Weight Loss Journey: Part Two

Reaching Goal, One Pound and Story at a Time

JORY AMES

Publisher: Wordsworth LLC Publishing
www.wordsworthwriting.net

To contact the publisher, e-mail: editor@wordsworthwriting.net. To contact the author, e-mail: joryames@gmail.com.
This book is not intended to take the place of medical advice from a trained medical professional.

DEDICATION

Thank you for joining me on my weight-loss journey. I feel like I know you. Maybe it's because I shared so much with you about myself in my first Weight Loss Journey book, and now this one. But it's also because I've been you. I've read hundreds of weight-loss books and stories, hoping for the inspiration and answer to my own struggle.

Eventually, the answer came, and it came through my journaling. I hope the answer comes for you too. Despite all the challenges I went through this year, I learned to live a healthy lifestyle – so completely different than the one I lived a year ago. I had no idea that my weight-loss journey would bring me not only a new body, but a new way of living. It was a nice discovery.

Sometimes, the joy is in the journey itself, not just in getting to the destination.

Most of all, I dedicate this book in memory of my beloved Chewie, whom I lost during these months, as you will see. I will miss her always. To a good dog and a better friend. I love you.

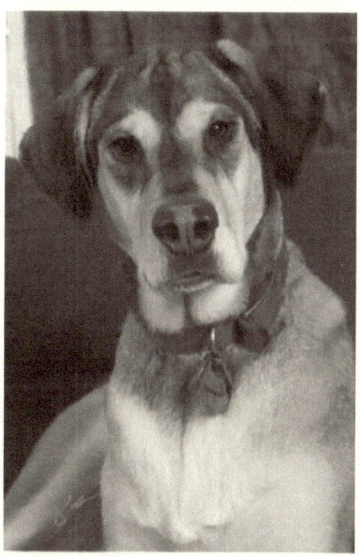

Photo of Chewie by David Jensen

INTRODUCTION

In her first weight loss book, Jory Ames set out on a journey to lose 50 pounds in 6 months. Her original goal and approach changed as she discovered the ease and comfort of living healthy.

This book is her journal to final goal, which was slightly less than she originally planned for but at the same time so much more than she hoped for or expected, all through healthy living. The changes in her life, appearance, and physical abilities are detailed through true stories and photographs.

On her way to goal, Jory faced obstacles, such as the physical pain of fibromyalgia, a sudden need for surgery, and the loss of her beloved older dog. She also quit smoking two months before this part of the journey, and she decides to add mental wellness to her journey, which leads (temporarily) to some unfortunate weight-causing medication. Incredibly, she faces a two-month weight-loss plateau, despite increasing her exercise. All these seem like roadblocks to achieving her goal. Still, she finds her way through without turning to food, as she always has before during life's trials.

In a year and half, Jory Ames lost 86 pounds. This final story is intended to be inspiring, entertaining, and even practical, as she details every inch, pound, calorie, and step.

CONTENTS

JULY 8-30

Weight: 161.9
Exercise: 5,000 to 10,000 steps a day average
Inches: Chest: 43.5 Waist: 36 Hips: 42
Body Fat %: 27.49% BMI: 27-4/5
Motivation: To turn my body into an athletic machine and never have to worry about being overweight again.

July 8, Wednesday

Weight: 161.6
Ate: 2 smoothies, 1 large bowl of beans with veggies and vegan sloppy joe mix, walnuts,
Exercise: Dog walk: 5,018 steps

And A New Journey Begins...

I feel like I'm beginning a new journey now.

My new journey is a healthy eating lifestyle instead of dieting. This is normal now. This is my new way of eating.

I feel freer. I am also surprisingly very full. Lots of veggies, beans, nuts, and fruit going in these last few days. I'm not worrying about amounts or calories. And I still lost another pound from yesterday.

Smoothie Ingredients

I generally stick with the same smoothie ingredients as before: a banana, seeds (sunflower or pumpkin usually), chocolate soy protein powder (for flavor), chia and flax seeds, spinach, strawberries, water, and ice. Lately, I have been experimenting with other choices. I like kale instead of spinach, as it makes the smoothies chewier (I put in the stems as well). I often change the fruit, such as using blueberries, mango, peaches, and others, usually frozen. I sometimes add half an avocado. Lately, I'm including oatmeal, just because of an accidental mixing of my sunflower seeds with oatmeal! I am slowly adding other vegetables, such as asparagus or carrots, as well as beans. It's not always a success and doesn't always taste good to me, but I'm learning to expand my vegetable choices.

July 9, Thursday

Weight: 162.5
Ate: Oatmeal, 2 smoothies, 1 vegan cookie, 2 big bowls of veggies with beans and Sloppy Joe mix, 8 crackers
Exercise: Dog walk: 10,750 steps

July 10, Friday

Weight: 164.5
Ate: 1 coffee with mocha; 1 giant bowl of veggies, beans, and vegan Sloppy Joe mix, walnuts, sunflower seeds, asparagus
Exercise: Dog walk: 12,674 steps

Eating "Normally"

Up 3 pounds; maybe eating "normally" is disastrous for me and "not an option." Rethinking this!

Perhaps I can never eat normally. You know what? I'm okay with that. I feel better (and look better) than I have in years. I have energy and even my concentration back (after losing it again when I quit smoking May 14). I'm good.

July 11, Saturday

Weight: 163
Ate: 2 Amy's frozen meals, 2 smoothies, beans, and asparagus
Exercise: Dog walk: 7,896 steps

Television Viewing

As part of my recently switching from Dish Network to Direct TV, I received all the movie channels free for 3 months. Unfortunately, going from "basic" Dish Network with only a few channels to hundreds of channels at the same price has caused my TV viewing time to increase dramatically. I would say I watch TV much more than the "average," which is shocking enough:

U.S. adults spend nearly 20 hours a week watching TV.
Fewer than half of them get the recommended 2.5 hours of

weekly moderate-intensity activity. (HBO. *The Quest...*)

For a few months, with only basic cable, I dropped my TV viewing down. Now, with the 3 months of extra channels, I have suddenly increased my viewing. What I see out there is almost nothing worth watching. But I am DVRing all the movies and documentaries I can in preparation for the long, dark winter ahead, like a squirrel collecting nuts.

Silly me. I think the DVR's role in America's fat epidemic should be considered!

Financially, being "stuck" with satellite for 2 to 3 years at a time per contract is awful, but I did it mainly so Greg could see football. We don't get any channels out here in the "sticks," and there's no cable offered here either. In Anchorage, when I didn't live with Greg, my son smartly figured out I could save $75/month by cancelling cable and buying streaming Netflix only ($8/month), which we did. That was a happy year TV-wise. Every night we watched an episode or two of *Lost* together; it was great fun and wonderful bonding time with my child; I was more productive without a DVR full of great things to watch, and I saved almost $1,000. Win-win-win! (However, I didn't lose a pound during that time. Those were what I call the "surgery years": four years of major surgeries: neck, both shoulders, knee, hysterectomy.)

July 12, Sunday

Weight: 161.9
Ate: Oatmeal with cinnamon, 2 slices of dry rye toast, ½ order of hash browns, 1 smoothie, ½ cup of walnuts, 1 large bowl of veggies with beans and sloppy joe mix
Exercise: Dog walk: 10,034 steps

HBO *Weight of the Nation* Series

Tonight, I watched a short film titled, *The Weight of the Nation: The Quest to Understand the Biology of Weight Loss.* (HBO Films). Here is how I summarized it to Greg:

"It was depressing watching this, because the [Columbia

University] scientists were basically saying people who lose weight are predestined to gain it back. Someone who loses 10% of their weight, and I lost much more, must eat 20% less or eat 10% less and exercise 10% more, the rest of their lives, just to maintain. The body and brain demand that the body goes back to the higher weight."

"Huh," the skinny little bastard said.

"They are experimenting with giving people the hormone leptin to battle this, but of course it's not something you can buy at the store or even get a prescription for."

"Huh."

"It was...well, discouraging."

We walked for a while, dogs running free around us, thinking about this.

"95% of the people who lose weight gain it back," I said.

"95?" he asked.

Yes, I was one of those. So many times, I thought to myself but didn't say out loud. Am I predestined to gain it back?

Depressing thought.

"Yes, 95%, and according to this program, the brain and body are making it happen."

I'm just talking it out, thinking about it. I come to a conclusion:

"What they didn't talk about much was people's food choices, especially processed foods and sugar. I think I'll be okay as long as I don't go back to those."

Then Greg started talking about the overweight construction workers he's worked alongside the last 30 years, and what was in their lunchboxes.

"I'd bring one sandwich, one carrot, an apple, a banana, and water. They'd have three sandwiches, candy, cookies, and soda. During our 10:00 break, I'd eat half my sandwich while they ate junk food."

"Yes, I see your point on food choices, but I can't disallow the role of hormones. If hormones weren't involved, then why did so many women gain so much weight when the birth control pill first came out?"

We walk in silence a little.

I then reiterate, "But I'm not going to gain this weight back. I'm going to be part of the 5%."

Let us pray.

Thinking about it later, researching what was said in this documentary online, I decide to see it as a way for these two researchers to get attention drawn to the possible role of leptin, but this is just a tiny piece of the weight-loss puzzle, and not one that will define me or determine my future. There are so many unanswered questions in it. As one online reviewer writes:

> *If the study was simply published in a journal and not projected onto a vast public stage such as HBO, there would less harm done.... This documentary perpetuated the myth of the almighty calorie while neglecting the importance of eating healthy foods, possibly exacerbating the obesity epidemic in this country.* [White Ink, IMDB]

July 13, Monday

Weight: 161.7
Ate: 1 Amy's frozen burrito, 1 giant bowl of veggies with beans and vegan sloppy joe mix, hummus with crackers
Exercise: Dog walk: 13,884 steps

10,000 Steps

Trying to make 10,000 steps my new "normal" every day, instead of the rare occurrence. Slowly, over the last six months, I've taken my daily average from the "red" on my pedometer program (less than 5,000) to the orange (over 5,000). Lately, I in am "in the green" most days (over 10,000). It's a struggle for someone who basically does not enjoy exercise, but it's necessary for a healthy, slim life. So it's what I do now. I accept it, not joyfully, but just accept it.

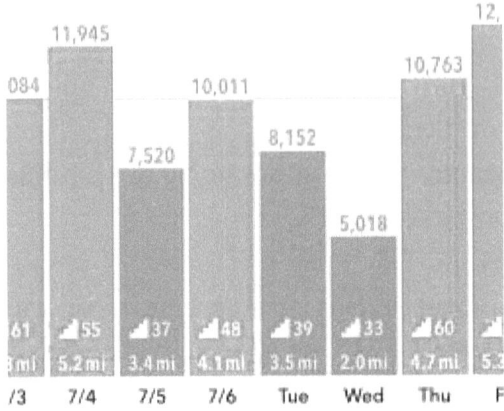

July 2015: Over 10,000 5 of 8 days. Over 5,000 all 8 days.

July 14, Tuesday

Weight: 162.7
Ate: 2 vegan cookies, 1 giant bowl of veggies with beans and vegan sloppy joe mix, hummus with crackers, 2 enchiladas with veggies, beans, and sloppy joe mix (yes, trying to use it up!)
Exercise: Dog walk: 7,363 steps

The End of the Contest

Today, at TOPS, for the first time 2015, I had a gain on the scale. My final competitor for the "Apron Contest," Janice, also gained (she 0.4; me 0.6). We agreed to a tie, happily, some sense of relief. Since January 7, we have motivated and challenged each other, being the last two names left on the apron for months, week after week losing weight. We joked about sending gifts of candy or cakes to each other's houses, but together, we inspired and battled with each other to lose a combined total of some 80 pounds. Good for us! It was a great run!

I celebrated the end of the contest by eating two vegan cookies; I think I've only had two in one day twice since starting my diet. I know that will probably be the last time in months I eat two of them in a week, but it was a special day, a final goodbye to the old me, and on with the new.

I suppose I should see the slight gain as a defeat of some sort, but I don't. I recognized it for what it was...salt. Last night I ate a large bowl of healthy but salty stew, and my body swelled up with the sudden influx of salt. it was bad timing on my part (the vegan sloppy joe mix, which I ordered, adds a great deal of taste to the beans and veggies I cooked, but it also is very high in salt, plus Greg added salt as well).

I'm not going to go crazy and give up and feel like a failure because I had my first gain of 2015 recorded at TOPS today. Somehow, instead, I feel more motivated than ever. I know that as I near my goal, I will see more bobbing up and down, and mentally I am prepared to take that in stride as necessary steps to my successful journey's end.

July 15, Wednesday

Weight: 163
Ate: 1 smoothie (added cooked beans and asparagus...not a good taste!), 1 Amy's frozen breakfast meal, hummus and crackers, 1 enchilada with beans and veggies
Exercise: Dog walk: 6,148 steps
Inches: Chest: 43.75 Waist: 36.75 Hips: 43
Body Fat %: 27.68 BMI: 28

The Dreaded Last 10 Pounds

So here I sit, back at 163, up 1.1 pounds from the start of July, over 2 weeks ago.

Oh, those last 10 to 15 pounds! How I hate them. Well, I don't hate *them*. What I hate is how much harder they are to lose.

But that's okay. Yesterday was my "free" day of eating vegan cookies and trying to "use up" the giant crock-pot of veggies, beans, and sloppy joe mix I made. I'm starting to think instead of eating the last two bowls, I should just toss it.

I certainly have that mental issue of not wanting to "waste" food, even though I'm still wasting it when I "hoard" the food as fat on my body. So, with the mental image of fat hoarding in my mind, I go into the refrigerator and cupboard and throw away food; some of it I give away.

Searching online regarding the last 10 pounds, I'm sad to say, many recommend weight lifting. "Sad" because I'm so bored at gyms. Sigh. But I put the weights and arm exercisers in my bedroom, so at least I can use those while watching TV. Currently, I do about half an hour of ab crunches while lying in bed at night. It won't be too much trouble to add arm exercises as well.

July 16, Thursday

Weight: 162.4
Ate: 1 coffee with cocoa powder and stevia, 1 Amy's frozen burrito, 1 smoothie, 1 Amy's frozen breakfast meal, 3 cups popcorn
Exercise: Dog walk: 16,252 steps

Slower Dog Walks

So Chewie grows old, faster than her sister does. Our dog walks get slower and slower, as she struggles to walk the trails, and needs plenty of water breaks. My exercise suffers for it, too, but that's okay. It's part of the beauty of having an old dog.

Chewie and her sister Blue ("Blue-Chew," Greg began calling them as puppies, and the combined name has stuck) both came to live with me 9½ years ago, as my first failed fostering attempt. (My second failure resulted in Kip and Harper moving in.)

The thing that's interesting about Chewie is her weight. She is heavy, about 108 pounds, definitely obese for a dog. She began gaining weight when she was a few years along in life. She eats the exact same as her sister (actually slightly less, for the last 5 years), goes on the same walks, does nothing different.

But she's fat. Blue is not.

There's an unfairness there. I think of the genetics research about obesity and wonder why they aren't the same, but then again, with dogs, there can be a different sire in the same litter. I think that is the case with Blue-Chew; Blue looks half husky and half German Shepherd; Chewie looks husky-Shepherd-hound dog-something else.

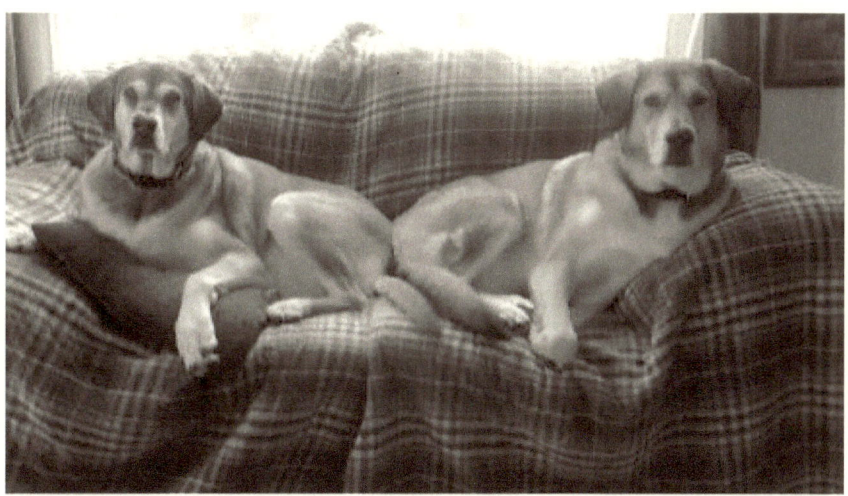

Chewie (left) and Blue (right) at about 7 years old. Phone by Jennifer Huntting.

I think Chewie's growing struggle to walk and the need for more water is surely related to her being heavier. Poor dog. I wonder if her obesity will kill her too early, and of course, I feel terribly about this, wondering what I could have done differently.

I don't think I could have done much.

I've had her thyroid checked, of course.

I've put her on weight-restrictive food. I exercise her daily.

She just, like so many of us, is prone to fat. I get that. I'm with her. As I fight to lose and keep fat off my own body, I watch her in empathy. I hang with her on the trails, while Greg and the other dogs run ahead. "I'm with you, girl," I say, patting her on the head, scratching her now-grey ears. "I understand."

More than anyone in this household, I understand. I know what it's like to have a body that can't seem to keep up...or to keep weight off. Of course, I fight my genetics, and I have no doubt I will win. But in the meantime, as I feel like I am growing younger and stronger in some magical way as my weight falls off (nearly 80 pounds since a year ago April), I watch my dog struggle and think, "I should have done more," and then think, "I am going to lose another great friend and soul soon."

Ah, the death of a dog breaks my heart in a thousand tiny pieces.

July 17, Friday

Weight: 162.1
Ate: Smoothie, Amy's frozen breakfast meal,
Exercise: Dog walk: about 4,000 steps (forgot pedometer), plus 2,956 steps on pedometer

The Latest *Dr. Oz Show* Diet: The Easy Summer Cleanse

The "big offenders" like "flour, dairy, sugar, and processed foods" have been eliminated from Dr. Oz's 5-day summer cleanse diet (sounds like mine, pretty much, except throw out meat too). Intended to last 5 days at a time, the first day includes juice with kale, fennel, parsley, lemon, green apple juice, and asparagus. Lunch is a smoothie of kale, avocado, coconut milk, dates, almond butter, and ice. Dinner is a smoothie with spinach, banana, sunflower seeds, and almond milk.

Wow! Sounds like my smoothies! I'm doing *awesome*!

Anyway, you can find Dr. Oz's 5-day cleanse diet at the link in the references (or just search online). The interesting part to me was the asparagus; supposedly, it helps your gastrointestinal (GI) system and helps eliminate bloating. Last week, I baked both green beans and asparagus, using them to munch on for snacks, so good to know. I might start tossing them in my smoothies.

The Day 2-4 choices include a lot of vegan choices, but also fish and chicken, so of course I would not eat those. But certainly it's a doable diet, if you're looking for one.

July 18, Saturday

Weight: 162.8
Ate: 2 smoothies, 1 bowl of oatmeal, 1 slice of toast, 1 vegan cookie, 1 Amy's frozen dinner
Exercise: Dog walk: 10,242 steps

The Internet

So my child, poor thing, has grown up in the Internet Age. He's had it worse than most, because his mother has worked at a computer every day, 7 days a week, for his entire life. When I'm not on the computer, I must check my phone, periodically, throughout the day and night, for online orders from a forms business. The Internet community demands that when something is purchased online, it is sent instantly, and the world is not always understanding when "instantly" takes an hour.

"Mommy, I had a dream last night," my son said, sleepy-headed and five years old, some 10 years ago. We'd fallen asleep in my bed reading books, talking, and watching movies. He woke up with his arms wrapped around my lab Buddy. Those two were always together, until Buddy passed away.

"What was your dream?" I asked.

"I dreamt," he said, looking up at me, "that you were saying, 'Because it's 5 a.m. in Alaska; that's why you don't have your form!' And you were mad!"

I laughed. "That wasn't a dream. Except the mad part. I wasn't mad."

"In my dream you were."

"Well, I wasn't. I would never be mean to a customer." I kept the phone next to my bed so I could answer the East Coast calls. Even though I had set up an automatic e-mail to all orderers explaining that we were in Alaska and didn't start sending till 5:30 a.m. (when Greg gets up and checks for orders) and stop sending at midnight, we'd still get the nasty calls sometimes. I always tried to be very polite and apologetic. I understand. You ordered it; you expect it now. That's the way the world is.

Sometimes I want to just shut down the forms business and unplug the Internet from my life. Go back to a cell phone that is just a phone instead of a "smart" phone. Especially now that the forms business has basically died. I still have to be on guard, to check for orders, night and day, yet I might only sell one form all day instead of 15 or 20.

But then I think of the 13 years I gave up of my life making those 13,000 forms, and I want to cry. I don't want to give up. I want to check the phone in hopes of finding an order.

But to shut down the Internet and close up shop when I have put so much time into those forms? I don't know....

Still, I am starting to think I need to let go. Because of my son.

My son is addicted to computer games.

I am not the only parent in this situation. It is getting worse every day. Games like Minecraft, which I call "Mind Crap" and his dad calls "Mind Crash." Yes, it's creative, it's social, it's whatever.

It's a waste of time and life. It's an addiction. Like sugar and chocolate and cigarettes. Like alcohol.

My sweet smart child, who tested in the highly advanced levels and genius IQ, has been lost in this game for the last 5 years, and it feels like there is nothing I can do about it.

But there is one thing.

I can unplug the Internet.

If it can save our son.

He will hate us for it, furiously, beyond everything. I fear this more than death itself. But someday, maybe when I'm gone, he'll realize I did it because I love him.

July 19, Sunday

Weight: 163.3
Ate: 1 Amy's frozen meal, 2 smoothies, ½ cup of seeds, 1 vegan cookie, coffee with mocha
Exercise: Dog walk: 7,465 steps

July 20, Monday

Weight: 162.5
Ate: 2 smoothies, 1 coffee, carrots with hummus, 1 Amy's frozen burrito
Exercise: Dog walk: 7,690 steps

Attitude Dancing

There's a song by Carly Simon called "Attitude Dancing." I'm making it my theme song for the next leg of my weight-loss journey. Lyrics include:

Cop a different pose

From the pose you're in

Shine a different attitude

From underneath your skin

Attitude dancing

Strut around the floor in a different attitude

...Don't be afraid to change your attitude

Attitude dancing

Free up your spirit with a new attitude

I am no longer a victim. I am no longer dependent on other's views of my body, my weight, my food and exercise choices, my *self*. I free my spirit.

I eat what I want to eat. I don't eat meat or dairy, which means no more of what has always been my favorite food – milk chocolate. And, for that matter, buttered popcorn.

But here's the attitude dancing: I don't see this is a "Oh woe is me, I can't have what I want to eat" mentality, but as a "Yay! I don't want them, don't miss them, don't need them!" I don't see "diet" as a negative or a temporary situation. I see it as the glorious, happy, and healthy lifestyle choice it is. And I see how many food choices I now have as especially positive.

July 21, Tuesday

Weight: 160.4
Ate: 2 smoothies, 1 coffee, 1.5 bowls of oatmeal with peanut butter and cocoa powder, 1 Amy's frozen dinner, 12 dark chocolate-covered almonds
Exercise: Dog walk: 6,502 steps

ADHD and Me

I received a lovely e-mail from a reader of my *Weight Loss Journey* (the first six months), and I was surprised when she wrote this:

> *I could tell you were an ADD'er within the first chapter. Takes one to know one. I just finished a book that says ADD is a gift. The leaders of the world are all ADD'ers, as well as all the creative people and the folks who get things DONE. The winners of the world!!*

Over the past few weeks, I had begun to realize, as I realized my physical health – through weight loss, exercise, and quitting smoking – had improved, it was time to address my mental health. They are all connected, after all, and my overeating, anxiety, excessive worrying, smoking, and disorganization (or attempt to "over organize"), and relationship issues are problems that were apparent as I journaled my weight loss...I guess not only obvious to me.

The realization that not only I, but readers, could "tell" my little attention deficit disorder (ADD) (also known as ADHD, but I'm not sure about the "hyperactivity" part for me; I'm pretty lazy) secret stunned me, and set me on a new journey, a new book, to understand and "fix" my ADD. It is amazing how one journey leads to another to another to another.... I never thought, for example, that when I started my weight loss journey I would also become a successful nonsmoker. I am excited by the thought that finally, after all these years, I might learn to better manage my ADD and reap the benefits of my newly found knowledge, just as I am enjoying my new physical health. Wish me luck!

July 22, Wednesday

Weight: 161
Ate: 2 smoothies, 1 coffee, 1.5 bowls of oatmeal with peanut butter and cocoa powder, 1 Amy's frozen dinner, 12 dark chocolate-covered almonds, 1 vegan cookie

Exercise: Dog walk: 5,071 steps

Oprah's 800-pound Man

I found some weight-loss success stories from an old (2003) Oprah show on On Demand, so I watched it. The women's stories of losing 100 to 200 pounds were inspiring. Most of them lost the weight within a year or two, all through diet and exercise. Then a man came out. He had weighed over 800 pounds. He had lost about 600 after weigh-loss surgery. He was happy, excited, able to get out of his house for the first time in years.

Here's the awful part. After his "little" story was done, there was a message on the screen that he passed away from congestive heart failure, in 2003, which means that same year.

NOOOOOO!

Not fair! Not right! No good! After all that tortuous surgery and dieting, and then he DIES?

Dang it.

Somehow, it made me think of my own heart. I never thought of the fat I was sending straight to it. I hope my heart lost weight along with the rest of me.

July 23, Thursday

Weight: 162.5
Ate: 2 Taco Bell burritos, 6 Amy's burritos, 1 smoothie
Exercise: Dog walk: 5,193 steps

Old Dogs and Short Walks

Ate a lot of burritos today! Hungry! Crazy day. Lots of errands. Short, easy dog walk today and yesterday due to Chewie's growing weakness. She has a vet appointment tomorrow, so here's hoping we can find something to help her. I just can't bear to leave her behind during the walks, but it's definitely slowing us all down.

Her sister, Blue, who will also (of course) be 10 years old in December, is the one I was always told wouldn't be able to walk past a year old, due to hip and elbow dysplasia. But she does fine.

The difference is their weight. Chewie is fat. And she's suffering. She struggles and rests frequently, wandering into the weeds. I feel badly about her weight. Somehow, like fat children, fat dogs seem like "mama's fault."

This morning, I heard a large crash in my bathroom; Chewie figured out how to open the cupboard door and knocked over the container containing dog food and was munching away at the giant mess she made. I cleaned up 50 pounds of dog food from my bathroom floor, or maybe 40 pounds after she was done ravaging it. Sigh.

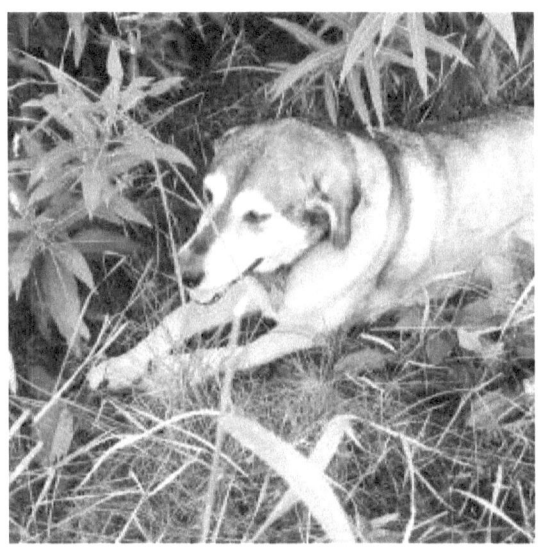

Chewie stopping to rest during our walk; this has never happened before.

July 24, Friday

Weight: 163.5
Ate: 2 smoothies, 1 Amy's burrito, 2 cups popcorn, ½ cup seeds, veggie burger, carrots, grapes, 1 vegan cookie
Exercise: Dog walk: 10,074 steps

Pants

This morning, walking the trails with the dogs earlier than usual (which seemed to help Chewie), my pants fell off! Literally!

I was alone with Greg and the five dogs in the Alaskan wilderness, so I didn't try to stop it from happening. Instead, I waited for it...waited...then felt them tumble down.

Yes!

That victory felt as marvelous as any of them, probably better. It was an actual proof of my hard work and strict attention to diet.

"I'm too small for stretch pants!" (at least XL stretch pants), I thought, happily. I pulled back up my pants, which I will never wear again, and happily walked home.

July 25, Saturday

Weight: 162.6
Ate: 1 Diet Pepsi, 1 coffee with mocha, 1 order of sweet potato French fries, 1 Amy's frozen burrito, 1 soup, 2 smoothies, 1 bowl of oatmeal with peanut butter and chocolate
Exercise: Dog walk: 2,956 steps

Lazy Day...

Only day this month I haven't achieved at least 5,000 steps. The dog walk was very short; I instead spent the morning riding with my son driving my car. What an experience! He drove me around Palmer.

First time ever that's happened.

I bit my lip and gave him the key, and he did great. Of course, he's had four driving lessons (so far), six to go, from a professional. Worth the $600 to get someone else to teach him. I've given him a few lessons in empty parking lots, but I was afraid to go on the roads till he had lessons.

He did great, even with the dogs going crazy in the back seat as they complained about not stopping for their walk.

I was able to manage my anxiety and worrying, praised him, bought him lunch, squeezed a short dog walk in between, and survived. Only slammed on my imaginary brakes once. And didn't turn to food. The "old me" would have been popping M&Ms in my mouth the entire hour or so. I'm not kidding.

July 26, Sunday

Weight: 161.7
Ate: 1 Amy's burrito, 2 bowls of oatmeal with peanut butter and chocolate, 2 smoothies, 1 coffee, 1 small Diet Coke, 1 cup of soup
Exercise: Dog walk: 6,776 steps

Hoarding and Obesity

Happy to make another bag of clothes for Goodwill. I am not replacing the clothes with new ones; instead, I am paring down. Yes, most of my clothes are now "too big," but I don't care. Much better to have them too big than too small! The main thing is, the more I clean out and get rid of "things," the more unstuffed I feel in my mind. I am loving the clean countertops and opened-up spaces in my house. I actually felt so happy walking into my bedroom today, all free from clutter. I am not alone. Per *HubPages* ("New Research..."):

> *Interestingly, a lot of obese women who have lost significant weight (30 pounds or more) stated that one of the first things they wanted to do as the weight started to fall off noticeably was not so much to buy new clothes, but to clean house!*
>
> *Yes, that's right, they reported a strong urge to purge the house of junk the same way they had purged their body of the fat, so this may actually be the key to controlling the defunct gene.*

I don't enjoy organizing, but I enjoy the results. I have noticed, as I've said before, that almost every person on the show *Hoarders* is heavy. So I look this up. It turns out some 92% of "high savers" are overweight or obese, which suggests "there may be an underlying genetic association with the dopamine system" (Helwick). As Jamie Feusner, MD, says:

> *"Clinically, our only explanation has been that hoarders are using food as a substitute for human relationships, since these are often lacking. We notice that they often develop*

emotional attachments to the objects they acquire. Food
may be a way of self-gratification and soothing...a genetic
association with the dopamine network, which is involved in
the reward system, would be interesting." (qtd. in Helwick)

July 27, Monday

Weight: 161.3
Ate: 1 Amy's breakfast, 1 cup sunflower seeds, smoothie, soup
Exercise: Dog walk: 5,650 steps

Dopamine and Obesity

Dopamine is a brain chemical that gives feelings of pleasure and satisfaction. The lack of or search for an increase in dopamine seems to be the key in many addictions, such as sugar, chocolate, cigarettes, alcohol, and overshopping or hoarding, as well as numerous drug addictions. I don't need a genetic test to tell me I'm seeking dopamine "hits" by shopping or eating candy and ice cream or smoking.

Or rather, I was. Now I'm using exercise to jolt my dopamine.

Brookhaven National Laboratory (BNL) writes that obese people have "fewer receptors for dopamine," suggesting that they might "eat more to try to stimulate the dopamine 'pleasure' circuits in the their brains, just as addicts do by taking drugs" ("Scientists Find..."). Interestingly, BNL tests showed that the higher a person's BMI (or the more obese), the fewer dopamine receptors she or he had.

So here's hoping I'm increasing my dopamine receptors by losing weight and exercising. You can also search the Internet for foods that might help dopamine levels; see for example Wylde's "The Dopamine Diet" (see References section). After reading it, especially since I have ADHD, I decided to try L-tyrosine supplements, so I'm placing an order for a vegetarian kind online. It's worth trying to see if it helps me feel better mentally.

July 28, Tuesday

Weight: 159.8
Ate: Veggie burger with small fries and Diet Coke, ½ cup of popcorn,
hummus with tortilla
Exercise: Dog walk: 6,064 steps

Into the 150s!

I only lost 0.6 pounds from last week's TOPS meeting, but I have to say that today's weigh-in felt better than any previous one ever. For I got into the 150s today! It's been 8 years since I've been here.

150s. Sigh. The 150s are where my body might "settle." I don't know. I'm just going to keep plugging away at my vegan diet and daily dog walks and see.

This is where I will achieve my healthwage.com goal (153) and win $800!

This is where I will perhaps reach KOPS status in TOPS; I say "perhaps" as I'm going to let my body decide when it's reached a comfortable set point, whether that is 153 or 145 or 140. I'm just along for the ride, enjoying every minute now.

Especially now that I'm in the 150s!

Today, I dropped off another contractor bag of too-large clothes at Goodwill, popped inside (which I usually don't do because I don't want more stuff), and bought myself four size-medium shirts. Medium! From XXL to M in seven months. I'll take it! I *love* the 150s!

July 29, Wednesday

Weight: 159.9
Ate: 1 Amy's frozen breakfast, 2 smoothies, 1 cup sunflower seeds
Exercise: Dog walk: 10,000 steps

Pain Update

In my first diet journey book, I wrote about the pain I live with daily, fibromyalgia. As I sit typing, I feel it constantly, today in my knees, shoulders, elbows, and hips, especially. So has losing 80 pounds helped? Has increasing my exercise and decreasing my time sitting at the computer reduced my pain levels?

I'd say, "probably yes," if you asked me that question. I was hoping, since it is summer (and the pain is worse when it's cold) and my being vegan (which seemed to help before), that I would have zero pain by now. I don't have that. But it's certainly bearable, and I haven't taken an actual prescription-strength pain pill for six months, which is awesome! I have taken two Advil-type pills all summer, and I used to take them daily, like vitamins. So the pain level is definitely much lower than it has been in at least eight years. I'm crediting the vegan diet and the flaxseed, as well as the lack of work and therefore fewer hours at the computer. And of course, most of the credit must go to the dogs, who force me to get up and walk every day.

It would be nice to have zero pain. That might never happen for me. Like all chronic pain sufferers, you learn to live with it, to deal, to accept. I know heating pads help, as well as Icy Hot or Ben Gay lotion, and hot baths. I just try to use treatments that aren't drugs. But still searching for the answer.

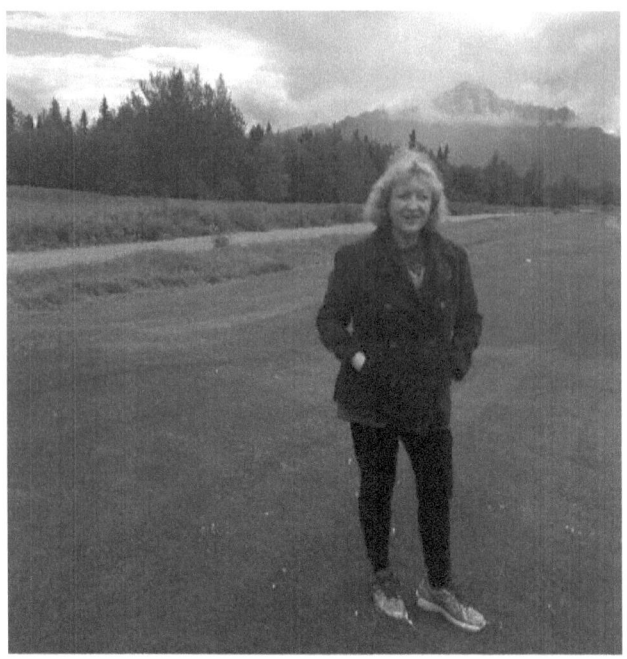

Today, while waiting for my son to try golfing for the first time. Nice mama to pay for it! I'm wearing a coat I haven't fit into for eight years (the only item of my "skinny clothes" I saved).

July 30, Thursday

Weight: 160.3
Ate: 3 burritos, 1 smoothie, 4 cups of popcorn
Exercise: Dog walk: 4,335 steps (shortened because Chewie was struggling)

Back up to the 160s (barely), but I know this is the typical bouncing up and down that mainly goes down. So I'm good.

July 31, Friday

Weight: 160.5
Ate: Amy's frozen breakfast meal, smoothie (new kind with 1 avocado, 1 banana, cocoa powder, and 2 packets of Stevia – consistency of pudding!), 1 can of soup, 1 large order of onion rings, 1 Diet Coke
Exercise: Dog walk: 11,142 steps

Ritalin

Today, I made some great progress on my third self-improvement project of the year: understanding and managing my attention deficit disorder (ADD). I have started a third self-help journal tracking my progress, the same as I did with my obesity and smoking.

I also tried Ritalin (actually the generic for it, something I've had sitting in my bathroom cupboard for four or five years, but have been afraid to try. It wasn't a terrific experience. I looked up (after I took it, of course, idiot) the side effects of Ritalin, and one possible side effect is weight loss.

"I'll take it!" I think, even though my brain feels funny and warm. Overweight women – or at least me – are so pathetic!

Of course, for some stupid reason – Ritalin? – today I ate the worst thing I've eaten since I started my weight loss journey: a large order of onion rings from Dairy Queen (yes, it was my day to take my son there, and for the first time, he *drove*!).

Why did I lose control eating? That's not like me, not like the new me anyway? It has to be the Ritalin! Dang. I suppose I'm going to be one of those rare people who gains instead of loses weight on the stuff. I found one site (ehealthme.com) that says only 2.98% of people gained weight on Ritalin, but interestingly, that goes up to 19.05% of people (like me) in the age 50-59 bracket. I check sites (such as talkaboutsleep.com), and some say their appetites were actually stimulated by Ritalin.

It is evening time, and I took my second pill. The first one made my head feel funny and led to tears; after the second one, my head feels fine, but I feel like my heart is going to explode since it is racing so much. (Maybe the nicotine gum didn't help?)

Sitting here scared, terrified of dying from medication that is supposed to make me better. Gag. Argh! Ugh!

Today was also the day I was headed to the Butte to climb it, something that has been on my "bucket list" all summer. But then Miza ruined it. Like he does so many things. And suddenly I realized: my dog has ADHD! Here's what I wrote; I thought you'd enjoy it.

My ADHD Dog

So, today was supposed to be the Big Day When Mom Achieves One of Her Goals for the Summer: Climbing the Butte in Palmer, Alaska.

I was only going to take the puppies, because the older dogs – Blue and Chewie – are having troubles with tough hikes these days, and Miza, well, he's Miza.

I manage to get the puppies downstairs and the door closed with the older three dogs upstairs, but my son lags behind.

When he opens the door, Miza, of course, comes bursting down in all his raging barking growling mess of madness.

Fudge.

Greg wants to know why we have three dogs going with us. What he really means, of course, is, "Why is Miza going?"

Now, Miza has gone on every hike with us for the last 6 years (feels like 20 or 30), but he is the worst dog in the world to travel in the car with. Especially if he doesn't have "his" seat...the front passenger seat. During the drive, he bounces back and forth, barking and growling furiously, terrorizing the puppies, jumping on me and scratching my legs with his 65 pounds of horror.

Miza is my least-favorite dog I've ever had. (Actually, I can't say I've ever really known a dog I didn't *like* before him. And I do love him. I just don't *like* certain parts of his personality.)

I knew within 10 minutes of taking him out of the pound that he was trouble, but I certainly wasn't taking him back.

He is an anxious, crazed, mouthy mess. He never settles down. He won't stop complaining.

He is me, in a dog. (How did I not realize that till now?)

Brat. Miza, you're a brat for being a mirror to my ADD face, only you are almost 100% the "H" (hyperactivity) in ADHD, so I'll use that term here.

I thought he'd settle down once he knew he was our forever dog. "We don't give dogs back," I'd say, scratching his silly black ears. "You can relax now." But he's crazed, in the brain, somewhere. Still, he's grateful, and he tries hard, but it's just not in him to relax.

I've even tried getting medication for him, brain drugs, like I am now trying for myself, but some kind of doggie downer in his case, "just so I can drive to Anchorage and back without him breaking my eardrums," I beg the vet.

The drugs made Miza furious. He seemed to know he was not himself, and he became even angrier in trying to stay connected to what he knew. It was kind of fascinating, actually, watching him fight the drugs that were supposed to mellow him and put him in a semi-trance. He was always victorious, coming out of the epic battle between Miza and Miza's-brain-on-drugs more cantankerous than ever. So, drug fail. I tried about three or four times and gave up (which is probably what I'll do with Ritalin).

There is no doubt Miza loves us, completely and fully and protectively, by the way. It's just that he's a little hard to be around sometimes. A lot hard.

In fact, today, after about 30 minutes of it, and Greg's complaining along with my own whining, I told Greg, "Just turn around." And he did. It's the first time in all these years we actually gave up before arriving at our destination with Miza. Maybe we're too old. Maybe it's my medication. But I couldn't stand one more minute of the furious leaping, jumping, whining, crying, barking, growling mess of a dog throwing himself around the van; herding the puppies to the back; jumping on me in the front; barking in my son's ears in the middle. I wonder if this is what my ADD makes others feel like.

I guess climbing the Butte will have to wait for another day. ADHD dog ruins it!

What I Did Right and Wrong This Month

What I have done right is:

- I lost 5 pounds this month, which is awesome, I believe, this far along in my journey (on July 1, as published in my first *Weight Loss Journey* book, I weighed 165.4). Mostly, I am happy with my attitude – being this ecstatic with a loss of "only" 5 pounds. Victory dance! Happy moves!

- I arrived into the 150s for the first time since 2008 (seven years ago)! My weight loss might "settle" into the 150s, or, perhaps (I hope?) the 140s. I don't know. I'm just going to continue eating right and exercising and see where this plane lands.

- I kept plugging away at the dog walks, missing none. Not one!

- At night, in bed, I would sometimes do sit-ups and leg lifts. A few times, I got out my weights and did arm exercises while watching TV.

- I made it at least 5,000 steps every day but two. I made it 10,000 steps 13 days.

- I began working on another issue, one that affects my health and relationships: ADD.

- I was much more active overall, actually going to a few community events such as the Fourth of July Parade and a Garden Festival. These things are hard for me to do, but I got out and did them.

- I didn't smoke one cigarette in July 2015! I have now reached 11 glorious smoke-free weeks! And yes, I still lost weight. Feeling proud of what seemed impossible.

- I never starved. I never went hungry. I relaxed and ate more some days this month than I did my entire previous six-month journey. I experimented with more food to see what I could consume during weight-loss maintenance. I didn't feel like I was in a hurry to lose "60 pounds in 6 months" as

I originally set out (and failed, although none of it feels like failure) to do. Now I'm just aiming to get healthier and fitter, that's all.

What I have done wrong is:

- Oh my Lord how I hate that I can't just get my butt in the car and drive to the gym and lift weights. What is wrong with me? It's paid for; it's not that far away; what is my problem? I pretty much know it's people, and my general loner mentality. *Need – to – work – on – this!*
- I avoided the treadmill. Per usual.

AUGUST

Weight: 160.8 pounds
Exercise: About 10,000 steps a day (dog walks)
Inches: Chest: 43.5 Waist: 36.5 Hips: 41.5
Body Fat %: 27.51 BMI: 27-3/5
Motivation: To reach my healthywage.com goal and get my hard-earned
money! To achieve KOPS status at last at TOPS, after some
14 years of trying.

August 1, Saturday

Weight: 160.8
Ate: 8-10 beans (baked with oil; salted); 2 smoothies
Exercise: Dog walk: 17,028 steps

Fitbits

Every once in a while someone invents something that just changes your life, or you feel like it can.

It was that way with the first computer. The home treadmill (which I don't use). The television (gosh, I'm not that old; what am I saying?). The free Pedometer app on my iPhone.

And now, the...drum roll please...Fitbit! (Once again, no companies have paid me for their product reviews!)

Yesterday, I tried out my new Fitbit. After some initial confusion (had to go online for the instructions) and some difficulty actually getting it to stay on my wrist, my phone and computer were synced and linked to my Fitbit. I am sure I will have more steps now that I don't have to carry my phone around with me to record them, plus it does awesome GPS tracking, shows mileage, calories burned, and has something in it that monitors my sleep!

Wow, what a brave new world! (I think I mean that in a good way?)

Anyway, I then posted on Facebook to people to try to connect with me through the Fitbit app, so we could challenge each other (as two women in TOPS are doing, which is where I heard about

Fitbits), and wouldn't you know my good ole healthy friend Cindy chimes in and says she's ordering a much better Fitbit than I have.

I ordered the Flex for $75, and it monitors not only my steps but my sleep. It is perfectly sized, like a woman's watch. But I was saddened that it didn't have the time or anything else on it, just lights. I have to check my steps, etc. on my phone.

Cindy ordered the Fitbit Surge for her and one for her husband. I guess they are richer than I am. I pouted after I read her post:

> *"I got the Fitbit Surge because it has a heart rate monitor and GPS tracker. Steps aren't enough for me. Chris and I run and need to know the distance and time. Other Fitbits don't measure that."*

So then I offered my Flex to Greg, and showed him what Cindy ordered and said I wanted this too. Of course, then Greg wanted the Surge also. So my little Facebook post ended up costing me $500. Fortunately, Amazon is taking back the Flex (I can't get my son interested in a Fitbit; I offered it to him). I have to say it's perfectly sized for me. I am hoping the Surge isn't too bulky. But I'm competitive, and I have a feeling this Fitbit thing, especially challenging Greg, Cindy, and Chris, is going to change my life for so much better.... Stepping into more than weight loss, but into fitness.

August 2, Sunday

Weight: 160.9
Ate: 2 smoothies, 2 Amy's frozen meals, ¼ cup cashews, 2 cups watermelon
Exercise: Dog walk: 15,178 steps

Hypothyroidism: Dogs and People

Two weeks ago I took Chewie to the vet. We ran a series of examinations and blood work. Even though I have had her thyroid checked before, and it came back normal, both the vet and I agreed it should be run again. This weight gain doesn't make sense.

"For the last three years, I have cut her food down more and more. She still goes on the same walks as the other dogs. But she is overweight, and they are not," I explained. She also gained another 10 pounds in the last year, an incredible amount of weight on a poor dog's heart and liver and joints. Probably equivalent to the damage 50 extra pounds was doing to my body.

Then I told how she is suddenly exhausted, thirsty, and slowing down and even stopping during our walks. So I spent the $500 for the thorough exam and blood work. My dogs are my family. What else is one to do?

An initial blood test showed (barely) low thyroid. Both the vet and I grinned in relief. Greg didn't understand. We explained it to him. My (long-deceased) dog Dane had hypothyroidism, and almost instantly after going on the medication, her energy levels increased, her hair grew back on her belly, and she lost weight. It was miraculous!

I am telling you this because sometimes weight issues are caused by thyroid issues, whether in dogs or humans. It's worth checking. In the case of hypothyroidism, there really is a magic pill. After the initial blood work was confirmed by blood tests performed by a laboratory, Chewie finally got to go on thyroid medication last week. I am so happy for her.

(Her blood test results put her in the absolute bottom of normal, which is where I always was too, so doctors therefore did not treat my hypothyroidism. But the veterinarian wanted to try medicine with Chewie, and I completely agree. If she gains any more weight, she won't be able to walk at all. I'm quite certain she needs thyroid medication. We agreed to try for six weeks, and then recheck her blood. Oh, if only medical doctors could be so simple to work with.)

August 3, Monday

Weight: 159.8
Ate: 2 smoothies, 1 can of soup, 1 Amy's frozen meal

Exercise: Dog walk: 10,707 steps

Fitbit Challenges

So my steps have increased dramatically the last 3 days since getting a Fitbit. Part of this is because I'm wearing it all the time, as opposed to carrying my iPhone pedometer with me. But mainly it's the challenges.

Last night I kept walking Kip, tossing balls for him, monitoring the progress of my three challengers on the Fitbit app on my phone. I walked up to first place by 6:30 p.m., but then Janice from TOPS (my former Apron contest competitor) passed me. Obviously, she was monitoring my steps too. "Good God, I concede at last!" I messaged her; it was already 2 hours past my usual wind-down and crawl in bed with the dogs time! What a great little "toy" this is, and finally, I can play a "game" that isn't a waste of time and life. Instead, this game will extend my life and improve my health.

Mondays and Weekly Weigh-ins

I don't go hungry much these days. I have found that good healthy foods – especially smoothies and soup – help me to feel full, or at least, not starving. (Before, I could eat 2 pounds of chocolate and still be ravenous.)

But there is one day a week where I might get hungry, trying especially not to snack. That is Mondays, because Tuesday mornings are TOPS weigh-ins.

The weekly weigh-in is the best part about going to a weight-loss group, in my opinion. It gives you a goal each week. Maybe you bounce up and down like I do every other day. But each week, I have a goal...to lose weight for the next TOPS meeting. It helps me have a steady loss. Even if that loss is "only" half a pound a week, in 52 weeks, or one year, you've lost 26 pounds! Think of lifting 26 pounds. That's a lot of weight on the knees, the joints, the back, the feet, the heart. Our beautiful, lovely, powerful hearts.

Let's love them back, as they love us, and lose a little weight.

August 4, Tuesday

Weight: 158.8
*Ate: 2 vegan wraps from Fred Meyer, nuts, 1 cup of chocolate-covered
almonds, 1 Amy's frozen burrito, 1 cup of soup*
Exercise: Dog walk: 13,897 steps

Crazy Day

Down a pound since last week's TOPS meeting. I'll take it!

Got a couple big projects (work! Yay!) today, but halfway
through, I actually forced myself up to walk the dogs on the trails.
Proud of that. But was not happy to see my puppy, Harper Lee,
running toward me with what looked like a decomposed human
hand in her mouth. That's a tough image to get rid of. I got her to
drop it, took the dogs home, called the police, sent them pictures,
they couldn't decide if it was human or animal (bear would be the
only choice, but there were no claws or fur), the policeman came
out and walked the trails with me and after a while, he decided,
"It's not human," and so he tossed it in the tall grass (using a
stick).

It was so frightening and disgusting, and I still wonder if it
was human. But I'll do you a favor and not put the picture in here.
You don't need that image in your mind!

Even if it was a bear, the "fingers" were exactly my size. I
wonder what happened to it. Does this mean there's a bigger bear
somewhere in the trails I walk? Oh well, I'm less frightened of
bears than serial killers, that's for sure. Bears make sense.

10 Percent

Sometimes, during my weight loss journey, I strived to lose
just 10% of my body weight. I read that just losing 10% of one's
fat has incredible health benefits. So when I weighed 240 pounds, I
could picture losing 24 pounds. It sounded like a lot of weight, but
doable. Possible.

When I weighed 200 pounds, I aimed for another 20 pounds, down to 180. When I weighed 180, I aimed for 18 more pounds. And so on.

Now that I'm down to 158.8, I think, 10% is 15 more pounds. I'm not sure I exactly need to lose 15 more pounds, to 143. It would be nice, but then, I'm 55 years old, not 20, 30, or even 39, like the last times I was able to achieve that weight. I found it difficult to maintain, requiring hours of exercise a day and a near-starvation diet.

But then again, I wasn't vegan. Perhaps my focus on organic eating will make it possible, even easier, to get that far.

Ten percent more. Do I dare aim for that?

August 5, Wednesday

Weight: 158.6
Ate: 2 smoothies, 1 Amy's frozen burrito, giant vegan chocolate-oatmeal cookie; "pudding" smoothie with 1.5 avocados, cocoa, Stevia, peanut butter; sunflower seeds, and protein powder.
Exercise: Dog walk: 13,174 steps

How to Move a Treadmill

In studying ADHD, I realized part of the reason I dread using the treadmill is because of its location, down in what I consider "Greg's space," and the clutter that is there, which I can't bear. I began reorganizing and making space for it in my living room. I finally convinced Greg that I need it moved for my mental health, and he stopped taking it as an insult.

It's not easy moving a treadmill. I was willing to hire a mover, but Greg said that would be silly. So instead it's taken 3 weeks to get this done. Saturday, we actually tried to move it, four of us, and it ended up being a disaster. We were stuck in the hallway going up the stairs. My sheetrock has holes in it, and the treadmill is back downstairs. I had to assert myself to make Greg cease and desist before he killed one of the two boys helping us. "I will hire a mover!" I said, he tried to argue, and I said, "It's over."

Sometimes, a woman's gotta be firm to save the family and home.

So did he listen? No, the next day, Monday, I heard strange noises downstairs. He wouldn't dare, I thought, but I knew he was doing it. So my son and I had to help Greg lift the heavy monster up the outside stairs, one at a time. I feared death or injury to my son. But we made it, and now the treadmill sits in my living room, unused. Poor Greg.

Ritalin Update

No way in heck. That stuff was awful! Heart pounding, headaches, anger – crazy pill! Tossed in the toilet and gone forever. (It also made me hungry, so if you're thinking about trying it for the weight loss effects, which some people actually do, reconsider, please.)

I will not use medication to "manage" my ADHD, but I will instead celebrate the great things about it that make me unique – my creativity, my spark, my sense of humor, my empathy, my hyper-focusing on work, my ability to handle numerous projects at once.

And I will educate myself (just as I have with weight loss and quitting smoking) to find strategies for handling the negative parts about having it – especially my inattentiveness when my family is communicating to me. I will not drug myself for my distraction.

I'm not even sure ADHD/ADD is a "problem"; I think of it is a gift, in a way, for all I do and accomplish...so much more than the average bear (right, Yogi?). I was trying Ritalin because my son and Greg get irritated with me for fading away when they are talking or for interrupting them. Well, I've been this way as long as they have both known me. Can't they deal? Stupid to think mommy has to go on drugs just so they won't get mad at me for not listening.

Of course, that's not the only issue, but I'll work on all of them without medication! I suppose the ones that bother me the most are misplacing things (mostly fixed by setting up bins and hangers); and being (1) late or missing appointments, (2) anxious and a worrier, (3) unable to relax, (4) unable to focus on certain things (to do list, lectures and meetings, novels, TV shows, exercise classes, telephone calls), (5) disruptive, interruptive, the jokester, and opinionated in conversation, and (6) forgetful. A lot to work on. Just like all the extra weight was. So I research, plan, apply solutions, deal. Such is life.

August 6, Thursday

Weight: 159.8
Ate: 2 smoothies, 1 coffee with mocha, ½ cup of seeds and nuts, Amy's frozen meal, carrots, ½ cup nuts, ¼ cup seeds
Exercise: 2 dog walks and 15 minutes treadmill: 13,528 steps

Say What?

Okay, McDougall's. I've been a fan of your vegan soups for years, and even posted a picture of them in my *Weight Loss Journey* (volume 1), but as I was taking a photo of the soup I just ate through my Fitbit app (which automatically calculates calories you ate!), I noticed Fitbit popped up and said I ate 100 calories.

"Wow, only 100 calories for a cup of soup? Nice!"

Fine print stupidity alert. The label says this little cup, about the size of my hand, is two servings. TWO! Jerks! Who is going to share a little cardboard cup of soup with someone else? Or split it into two meals? I actually drank it all down in about one swallow. Ridiculous. *Stop doing that, stupid companies!* No wonder we're fat!

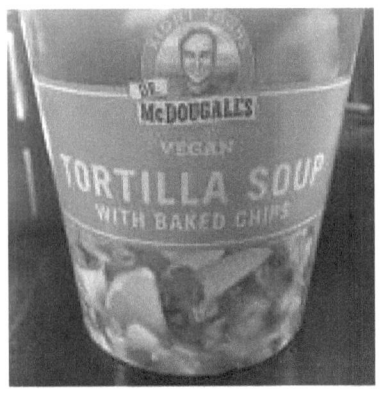 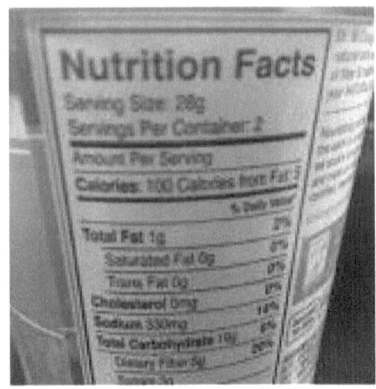

Smoothie Variations

Last night I invented a new smoothie; it tasted like heaven. Of course, it made for late-night eating and probably the (temporary, we'll hope!) pound gained. It included 1.5 avocados, chocolate protein powder, peanut butter, cocoa powder, and stevia, blended with ice and water. Yum. (I could have just used the protein powder instead of cocoa and stevia, but I didn't figure this out first try.)

For my morning smoothies, since passing the six-month mark on my weight-loss journey, I've been experimenting with the smoothie recipes. I've been incorporating a lot more vegetables and fresh fruits, for example. I keep my old standby of chocolate powder, flaxseed flakes, chia seeds, a banana, and a few frozen strawberries, but then I vary what I add, including some or all of the following:

- Raw nuts (cashews, almonds) or seeds (pumpkin, sunflower)
- Mangos
- Carrots
- Lettuce
- Sprouts
- Watermelon and other melon types
- Avocado

- Broccoli
- Cauliflower
- Berries of all kinds

I can't say there is one thing in this list above that I ever ate or liked before this diet (or life change). Maybe watermelon, once a year. But now I like them all – except berries. Not a fan of most berries except strawberries.

But that's not the point. The point is that I eat them anyway! Because they are good for my body and my mind!

Fat, Sick & Nearly Dead Documentaries

I am inspired by the documentaries *Fat, Sick & Nearly Dead* and *Fat, Sick & Nearly Dead 2* to put more vegetables in my smoothies, although I can't seem to convince myself to make juices (isn't all the pulp the most nutritious stuff?) or a juice fast, as advocated in the films. But I started throwing more veggies in my smoothies after watching the second one.

My brother gave me a juicer, which I haven't tried yet. I've never been a fan of juice in the first place, but secondly, I love my smoothies and they are working. I love the thick tough texture of them, and how I am basically "chewing" them. I love the cold milkshake feel of them.

And yet. Joe Gross, the films' creator and star, has inspired many to lose weight and get healthy through juicing. So it's worth a look and consideration. He has a website, rebootwithjoe.com, subtitled "Juicing for weight loss with Joe Cross." Ironically, the first thing that pops up at the top of the site is fattening fried chicken for a Popeye's coupon (pictured below).

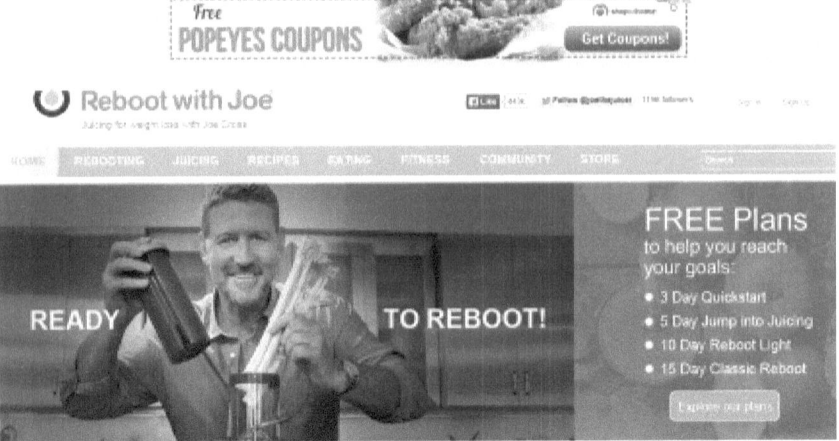

I know the guy's gotta make a living, but that seems odd. In any case, it's worth checking out the movies and the site, as well as considering trying juicing. The site also offers free guides and paid guided 15- or 30-day "reboots," currently ranging in price from $149 to $289. It's probably well worth it. Honestly, if I wasn't so far in my (successful) weight-loss journey, I might consider it. I did want to present it to my readers, as part of my reviews of books, movies, and websites.

But let me offer Joe's words here; certainly, I agree with the vegan diet (which seems to be what he's doing) idea:

> *"I am a much happier and healthier person since adopting a plant based diet that fuels my body with the nutrients it needs. My weight is steady, I'm off all prescription drugs and I rarely get sick."* – Joe Gross, "Guided Reboot.")

Thanks, Joe, for the entertaining and inspiring documentaries about weight loss. I wish him luck in his journey. My vegan diet seems a lot easier, but then I didn't have a disease to overcome like Joe did, fortunately. In the first movie, pictured below at left, he detailed how he went on a juice fast for 60 days to lose weight, get off pills, and get healthy.

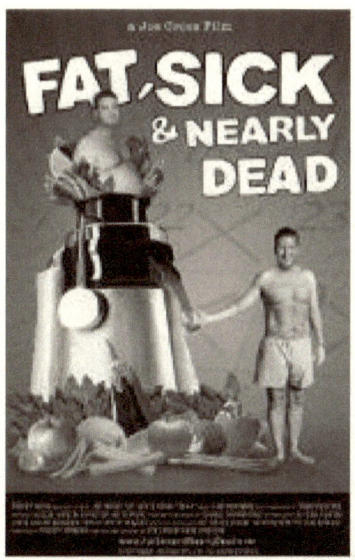 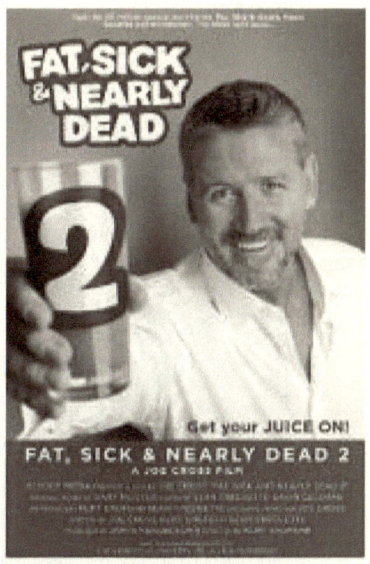

August 7, Friday

Weight: 158.6
Ate: 3 smoothies (including one "pudding" one with chocolate protein powder, avocado, peanut butter, kale, and sunflower seeds – yummy!), 2 sips of Diet Coke, 1 coffee (no mocha!),
Exercise: Dog walk: 13,865 steps

5 Pounds to Go to the $!

Five more pounds and I'll win the healthywage.com money! Almost there…. Can feel it…

Will I stop at 153.6? No. I need a good 10+ pounds more off my belly to be in the healthiest shape for my heart, knees, joints, and more. I'm aiming for the mid-140s. Happy dance. Before, I didn't allow myself to even dream I'd be back to the 140s after getting pregnant when I was 39, 16 long, fat years ago. But now I'm sure I will! It's nice feeling positive. This lifestyle change rocks!

My *Weight Loss Journey* (volume 1) book arrived in the mail today. Sigh. Here is the proud author (and thank you for reading!):

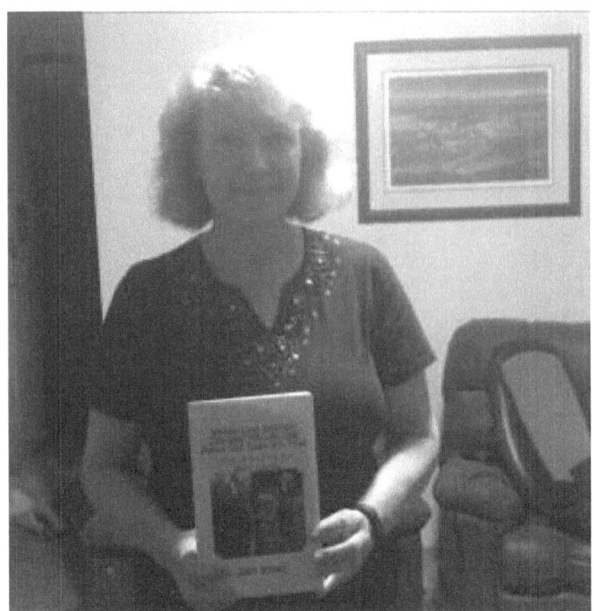

Fitbit Monsters!

My friends, all women about the same age as I am, none professional athletes, are Fitbit monsters! I think I'm amazing to get 10,000 steps a day; for them, it's normal to get 20,000 or even 30,000 or more! I can't believe it!

I don't know if it's the Fitbit competition (I think so), but it is astonishing to watch their progress. One of them, P, nearly always wins. She has all the excuses in the world not to work out. First, she lives in Louisiana, where it's been about 100 degrees every day this summer. Second, she has hives, which make her miserable.

P and I met at TOPS many years ago, had a close friendship, then spats where we didn't talk for months or years, then we'd reconnect. Now she's whipping me on Fitbit, getting me back.

The interesting thing is we've always been exactly in sync in our weight. If I weighed 220, so did P. If I weighed 180, so did P!

So this time, when we finally started texting each other again, 3 months ago when I weighed 172, after 3 years of silence, I knew she'd still be well over 200 pounds, so we'd finally be "unlinked."

Wrong! P weighed exactly 172! Strange!

Turns out she has diabetes now, and so she's been on insulin and the diabetic diet, and lost weight.

Oh. Sorry P. That could have been me, too. I'm so glad I lost the weight before I got that disease. At least we're not linked there.

So now I watch her Fitbit progress, proud of her, as she passes 30,000 steps most days. P rocks! She's an athlete, in my view.

Chewie's Thyroid

My dog's thyroid medication seems to be working; after just two weeks she has gone from 108 to 99 pounds, I'm happy to say. She still seems agonizingly slow on our walks, but this morning she made it the full loop, about a 3-mile walk, and I didn't have to turn around, so that's good. Whatever she needs, I will provide. I love old dogs. There is such a sweet sadness to them. The sweetness is theirs; the sadness is mine.... Dogs grow old too fast. (Except Miza, the brat ADHD dog. Kidding!)

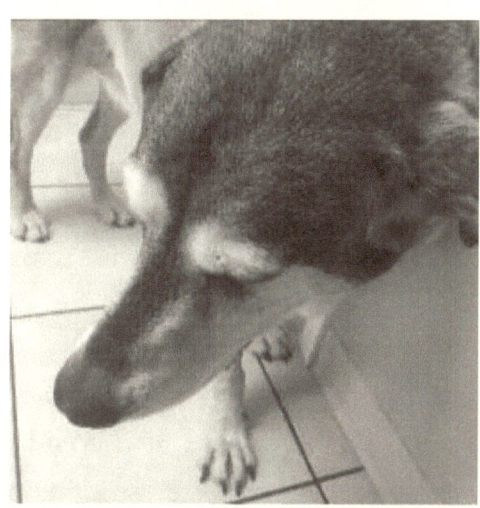

Diet Cokes and Pepsis, Oh My

Wow. On the way to the vet appointment today, I grabbed a Diet Coke from Greg's refrigerator. It's been days since I had one, but I think that might have been my last one. I could only stand two sips.

First, they are unhealthy; second, I don't even "like" the taste of them anymore. I guess my taste buds have changed along with everything else. Mostly, I just drank them out of habit, like smoking. Every morning, for the last 35 years at least, as part of my routine, I'd get a 32-ounce diet soda, filling my cup with ice first. That's 12,775 diet sodas. That's $12,775 at least, since the cost is $1.00 if I bring my own cup.

Bye bye, Miss American Sodas. I don't need ya, don't want ya, won't have ya anymore. Now, back to a nice cold glass of ice water! And it's free!

The amazing part about all this is, of course, how something so ingrained as a habit, such as drinking a soda a day, or eating M&Ms and Hershey's Kisses while working, or smoking to relieve stress, can actually be over, done, finished. I would never have thought it was possible for me.

Instead, I dropped into Fred Meyer and picked up a "Superfood Wrap" at the deli, which includes fresh veggies and hummus in a spinach wrap. Yum, and healthy!

August 8, Saturday

Weight: 159.2
Ate: 2 smoothies, 1 order of hash browns, 1 French fry (small; stole one of my son's), coffee,
Exercise: Dog walk: 17,273 steps

Expecting a Sudden Weight Loss

I don't know why, exactly, but I have a feeling my body is about to drop several pounds at once. I've been bouncing around the high 150s for a while, yet I've increased my exercise; in fact, I've about doubled my steps from my "normal" before the Fitbit arrived 9 days ago. I know I'm losing inches because all my clothes are much looser, especially the DG2 jeans I ordered in June; the size 10s are surprisingly baggy now for stretch jeans. I need to replace them with size 8s already, but I will wait another month or so and possibly order 6s instead, so I can wear them for years to come. Awesome!

Don't you love that feeling when you know you're about to have a nice loss? It's encouraging! It rarely happens, but once in a while I just feel my body is undergoing a muscular change, getting slimmer and tauter somehow. I'll take it! I deserve it.

Teaching the Feet to Jog?

A couple weeks ago I tried to run. I told my feet, run instead of walk, and then I watched them curiously as they stumbled awkwardly in the sand, not having any idea how to do what they were told. Like toddlers told to clean their rooms.

Odd. I forgot how to run!

I think back on childhood. How I loved to run. Just get my dog, disappear into the woods near our home (which are now long developed into college buildings), and start running. I ran for the love of the feel of it, for the stress relief it gave me, for the fitness, and to escape teenage woes.

I haven't run for at least 16 years, before I was pregnant, probably long before that. The knee injury and failed surgery after giving birth assured me my legs would never jog again. I could hardly walk without falling.

But that knee has been fixed now.

I just need to retrain my legs and feet to run again.

August 9, Sunday

Weight: 158.2
Ate: 2 smoothies, 2 Amy's frozen dinners, ½ cup nuts, hummus and chips
Exercise: Dog walk: 12,707 steps

Getting Motivated to Exercise

Yes, I've lost a tremendous amount of weight, showed incredible discipline, whatever, yada yada yada.

But I'm still lazy.

I take my dogs on a walk every day, sure, but I couldn't seem to get up to 10,000 steps daily until I got a Fitbit (which might mean I'm exercising more, but probably means I just wear it all the time, and I didn't carry my phone pedometer all the time).

But seeing how my friends are doing on the Fitbit challenges compared to me is pretty shocking. I'm last place nearly every day. By the time I wake up, Cindy (East Coast, 4 hours ahead) is well over 10,000 steps, and P (Louisiana; 3 hours ahead) is at 12,000. My TOPS nemesis, Janice, has already been out to feed the cows and pick up the grandchildren or whatever, and has logged 5,000 steps by 9 a.m.

Good Lord.

I need some motivation.

At This Rate...

At this slow rate of weight loss, about a pound a week, it will take me another 13 weeks to get to 145, where I want to be. That will be Sunday, November 8.

That seems slow, but I'm okay with that. I'm not starving; I can live with this way of eating for life; I am still moving every day, so I'm okay. I feel healthy and strong.

Of course, I'd rather lose the 13 pounds by tomorrow.

There's always that attitude.

But life goes on, and I'm enjoying the process, happy that I will be at goal weight in 2015. I'll take a pound a week. (But yay if it goes off a little quicker, anyway! We can hope!)

August 10, Monday

Weight: 158.3
Ate: 1 smoothie, Garden burger with veggies and ½ French fries and ½ onion rings; ¼ cup of seeds and nuts; 10 fresh beans with hummus, bowl of stir-fry veggies (no oil)
Exercise: Dog walk: 8,192 steps

Goodbye, Mr. Chips

So one thing I've been avoiding, generally (not mandatory like meat and dairy), during this diet is chips. It's not that I forbid them or haven't eaten them at all...if they are part of a meal I've ordered, I'll have some. I try to limit it to a small bag (such as baked chips when getting a Subway sandwich). But I don't buy them for my cupboard. Like salted nuts, they are too tempting for me to dive into, and let's face it, we all know there's not much nutrition but some extra pounds in a bag of chips, right?

So last night, after puppy class, I offered to stop at Walmart and let my son get some fries and a McFlurry at McDonald's. It's something I haven't done in probably the entire 8 months of this weight loss journey. He was so happy.

I said, "I'll be over here when you're done," motioning toward the deli section next to McDonald's.

Then I looked through the cases of the deli for something healthy I could eat, like the Superfood Wraps that Fred Meyer sells. But I found nothing but fattening foods or meat sandwiches, things like mozzarella sticks and jo-jos and cheese-bean burritos, all deep fried and disgusting, all things I used to eat as a vegetarian but never will again (both since I'm vegan and now eating healthy foods). So, finally, I found a container of hummus, and I grabbed that. Now I needed something to dip into the hummus; I looked through the breads and found nothing healthy. Just white and French breads and rolls. Awful choices! Eventually, I found a bag of large chips, checked the ingredients to be sure it was vegan, noted the oil (yuck), and grabbed it.

On the way home, while my son ate fries and ice cream, I had chips with hummus. Not a fantastic choice, but a better one than I could have done, considering the options. Thinking back, I realize I should have gotten celery or carrots to use for the hummus-dipping operation and eaten away without guilt, plus gained good nutrition.

The chips were yummy, crunchy, and addicting, so when I got home, I gave eight of them (they are huge) to the dogs, then took the rest down to Greg, my junk food garbage can, and said goodbye to them forever.

Sort of a win; sort of a fail. Next time, I'll definitely go for the veggies instead. Eating healthy is not always easy, but in this case, I didn't even consider the obvious choice.

The Scary Part: Studying Nutrition

You know me; I'm an anxious worrier.

So, the scary part about educating myself about nutrition has to do with my son. The kid who lives off cheese pizza mainly, grilled cheese and fries, McFlurries or Blizzards, and, rarely, some fruits. (Since I quit buying milk and rarely buy him juice, I've noticed he's increased his water intake and has slimmed down a lot.)

God, it scares me to death, what he's doing to his body.

Poor kid.

Bad mama.

Shit.

(Just now, I took action after writing that, and cut him up various kinds of fruit and put them in front of him, where he lives at his computer. Next time I checked, he had eaten them. Yay!)

August 11, Tuesday

Weight: 159.2
Ate: 2 smoothies, coffee with mocha, oatmeal with cocoa and peanut butter, pea soup with big bowl of veggies
Exercise: Dog walk: 10,262 steps

Reassessing the Diet

A few negatives to consider today. First is, bummerama, I gained 0.4 at the TOPS meeting compared to last week. Only the second time I gained this year for the weekly TOPS weigh-in (although it would have been three if I made it there the first week I quit smoking).

Second, yesterday I didn't make 10,000 steps, the first time since I got the Fitbit (and first time in August). However, I did accomplish a lot work-wise, and got caught up with some huge paperwork issues, so I suppose it's good to have those done.

So, time to reassess. Weight gain plus not exercising enough = Big Trouble in Little Alaska for Formerly Huge Woman.

I must catch it now, right here, at the start of the gain, before going back to the 160s, heaven forbid. I sit here, early evening time, and realize, okay, I got this. I know what I have to do. I don't want to, but I need to. I need to take control of myself.

This means a few days of restricted eating (dieting), focusing mainly on soups and/or smoothies. A soup or juice fast, so to speak. It's not going to be fun; I'm not looking forward to it, but I know it works, and it's always an option in case of a gain or in need of a quicker loss.

But, oh, how I still dread the hunger games days ahead. I like *not* being hungry. I have enjoyed the last 34 days of the "no-diet" diet; however, considering today's gain, I have only lost 2 pounds in all that time. (Still, losing ½ a pound a week is not bad, considering I tossed the idea of dieting, I suppose.)

And despite my attempts to find motivation, I am still, at heart, fundamentally, lazy. I don't find joy in the thought of exercise yet. I hope to get there, but instead of reaching for it, working at it, forcing it…I just wait for the exercise-brain to somehow find me and soak into me, becoming part of my being, like my diet has. I think it's going to take some research and effort to change this old-lady attitude into an athletic superstar!

August 12, Wednesday

Weight: 160.5
Ate: 4 smoothies
Exercise: Dog walk: 7,386 steps

Weight Loss Not

Spent all day caring for my son; he's sick, feverish, unable to eat, vomiting.

"I lost 5 pounds," he said, after one day of the horrible virus while we waited to see a doctor.

My instant reaction: "How do I catch it?"

In poor taste. Stupid. Regretted opening my mouth.

"Just kidding," I said. "I'm sorry," I added.

He just nodded, too sick to care about his mother's Big Fat Mouth.

It will be a few days locked in the house, sneaking out for a dog walk here and there, soft days full of worry and yet also no pressure to do anything or go anywhere, just hanging out near him, watching him, caring for him.

August 13, Thursday

Weight: 158.5
Ate: 4 smoothies; 1 can of soup; 1 bowl of vegetables, 4 crackers
Exercise: 2 dog walks 13,054 steps

Motto

Well, that worked, having a smoothie day yesterday. Two pounds back down. Yay! Catch it quick and take it down; that's my new motto.

(My old motto was, "Dang, I'm up again; oh well, I my as well keep eating. I can never lose.")

It was good to make it through a smoothie-only day. Not only did I lose 2 pounds, but I got my confidence back.

"I can do this," I thought today, happily putting more too-large clothes in another Goodwill bag. "I will make it to goal, and soon."

It was a good thought. The gain at this week's TOPS meeting kind of shocked me and made me afraid I was going to go back up, as I have in the past, every time I reached the mid-150s.

Not this time. Not – this – dang – time. I won't let it happen.

August 14, Friday

Weight: 157.8
Ate: Smoothie, oatmeal with cinnamon, ¼ cup nuts, 1.5 pieces of rye toast
Exercise: 2 dog walks 15,851 steps

Weight-Loss Surgery

One of the TOPS members had weight loss surgery a year ago, and she's lost about 170 pounds. Very impressive numbers, whether or not you had surgery! Wow!

She teared telling her story. I could read all the wounds she'd endured year after year of being the fat girl in those tears. I wanted to reach across the room and hug her and say I'm sorry for the stupid words from stupid people.

I wished I could have weight loss surgery. I loved the idea that I would never have to worry about fat again, and I could just get on with my life and living and being, without "I'm fat" being the loudest voice in my busy little brain.

"I'm fat" meaning "I'm not good enough," "I'm a failure," "I'm sad," "I'm miserable," "People don't like me," and "I can't."

Twice I called the doctor's office in Anchorage that performs the surgery, but they had a very complicated form that needed to be filled out by "your personal physician."

I don't really have one of those. I tried to think of who I could ask to fill it out. My brother? He would never understand.

"Eat less. Exercise more," he'd say, appalled.

"But I'm always hungry," I'd argue with him, in my mind, "and I work out every day walking the dogs! I *can't* lose weight! I've tried 1,000 times!" I'd be filled with protests and excuses.

The point is, the weight loss surgery would have helped. It would have been a relief.

But here's an even better point: I get the same relief, confidence, and assurance that I'll never be fat again as I would have with weight loss surgery from going vegan. For me, personally, it takes away all the fattening food choices. And I don't have the various health problems caused by the surgery that my sister does.

I feel golden, happy, good to go.

Maybe I don't have to hide anymore from people who knew me.

Maybe I'll age with grace instead of like a giant blob. Maybe I will still be walking when I'm 70 or – God forbid – 80.

(Will they serve me vegan food in the old-age home? I'm fretting about this already. My son better bring me food!)

August 15, Saturday

Weight: 157.1
Ate: 1 smoothie, ½ cup dark chocolate covered almonds, 1 Superfood
burrito (hummus and veggies)
Exercise: 4 dog walks: 24,291 steps
Inches: Chest: 41.5 Waist: 37 Hips: 42
Body Fat %: 27.66 BMI: 27

Shrinking Violet (i.e., Mae or Marilyn)

I guess the good news about my measurements is that my chest size dropped 2 inches since 2 weeks ago. I'll take it. The disadvantage to a large chest, as many women know, is back pain. For some reason, it's been one of the last places for the weight to disappear from, so I'm glad to see some go from there. Now I'll be happy to see the next 10 pounds come off the stomach and lower back – my middle. The fat sits there, but oh so much less of it than at the beginning of this year. There are so many reasons it is more comfortable being this way, one of which is I can't feel my stomach on my thighs anymore when I type. It's gone, girl!

Fitbit Fit

Three dog walks today. Exhausted and stressed, instead of what I should be: relaxed and proud. Happily tired. Not. Tired yes. Happy? No!

Why?

Gregory.

The Skinny Little Bastard is whipping me on Fitbit like crazy, and it infuriates me. I know I'm being childish and unfair. But it irks me how when I'm in the lead, he has to sneak out of the house, like a man with a secret lover, to go out for a run. Just so he can gleefully rub it in my face that he's better than me! And he goes without taking a puppy!

Without a puppy is what pissed me off the most. "Why can't you take one puppy?" I ask him.

He is furious. I have no right to expect him to do that.

He's right, of course. I'm the one who has dogs. Five dogs. Five. Dogs.

I'm the one who joked to a guy on the trails the other day, "Maybe I'm just too old for them," after praising him for his well-behaved dogs who ignored my puppies running toward them like manic clowns. And I was stunned when he agreed with me.

Doesn't matter if I'm too old for them, I thought, I have rescued them, and they are mine for their entire lives. But I'm 55 now, and by the time Kip and Harper Lee pass on, I will be past retirement age. These are probably my last puppies. The thought stings my heart, but for the first time in my life, I have to consider the end of my life, and how much my body can take, and most of all, the thought of dying before my dogs do. I can't trust what would happen to them without me, even though I tried to pull a Leona Helmsley in my will to make sure my pets would be cared for (my lawyer refused to do it!).

Of course, the puppies have made me young again, too. Would I be down 83 pounds now if I hadn't adopted them, or up another 20 or 30? I think I know. Those first 3 weeks of fostering six puppies, I lost 13 pounds. It was a miracle. I didn't know it was possible. It was all exercise...no diet. But I had hope now, something I had not had in at least 7 years of fat piled on fat.

Now, I'm a Fitbit athlete, pissed off because the Skinny OLD Little Bastard (14 years older than me!) keeps whooping my ass. But our Fitbit War has me going, walking, determined, angry, whatever. The dogs are getting slimmer, at least.

And Greg? I think he should consider the dogs as part of our family and want to help in with the puppy training so that these potential monsters learn some manners. I think my son should want to walk "his" dog, Harper Lee, since I'm paying a small fortune for them to take classes together. But no, once again, I'm alone with all this, just me and my dogs, as it's always been, and always will be, to the end.

I am blessed to have five dogs. That is my mantra. I must remember it, always. Even when the Skinny Little Bastard has over 20,000 steps to my 12,000.

Later: So my friends Bonnie and Jack dropped by to take their dogs for a walk. I waved out, saying I was too exhausted and had already taken three today, a record for me! They offered to take Blue and Harper Lee along, which was amazing – it was a puppy's first invite. Usually, they forbid the puppies to go with us on the walks because of their bad behavior toward their sweet dogs: barking, harassing, even – in the case of Kip – diving in and grabbing fur from their long-haired retriever.

So, I waved goodbye to Harper Lee, off on her first walk without me, on a leash, which I required through the parking lot. A few minutes later I receive a call from Jack. He took Harper off the leash, and she ran for home.

"I'll be right there," I said. I found my shoes and headed out, putting Kip on a leash to go with me. Greg followed, but, he told me later, "I left my Fitbit at home."

"Ah, you felt sorry for me!" I said.

"I didn't want your wrath," he grumbled, but smiling.

The best part of the walk wasn't getting over 24,000 steps for the day, my personal record. The best part was that I let Kip and

Harper off leash, and they were wonderful. Okay, there was one small mouthful of hair that Kip collected about halfway through, but other than that, they were angels: obedient, stayed close, nice to the other dogs. They both listened to me, watched me, respected me, loved me. Kip and I, in particular, have a special bond, that powerful rope of dog-human love that gets stronger every day. The "shy guy" is coming out, trusting me and my decisions, open to the world I present to him, letting go of his terror. Oh please, let it be true. I still have the marks of his terror on my thigh from the day I took him to a dog park. Maybe someday I can take him back there, and he will be fine.

I fell asleep the happiest I had been in months, thinking maybe my puppies wouldn't be worries to me for their entire lives! Maybe I can walk without fearing animal control taking my puppies or someone suing me because they attacked their dog. Maybe I can replace the horrible image of an old lady crying while Kip snapped at her older beagle with one of her smiling while the puppies sniff a polite hello. Maybe there is hope.

Of course, Kip snuggled in my arms for the night, tired and proud, sleeping deeply. I thought of how he was born, a year ago, in a pile of tires near Big Lake, along with five other puppies, raised by his mother, and no connection to people until animal control took them and caged them for a month before passing them to me, and how beyond frightened he was. How I worked extra hard with him because he shook so hard and tried to hide from people. And how he came to trust me.

I am a woman completely in love with a little black pile of fur.

August 16, Sunday

Weight: 156.5
Ate: 2 smoothies, 1 Amy's burrito, 1 large bowl of eggplant parmesan (minus the cheese!), 1 soup, ¼ cup of seeds, 2 smoothies, 1 Amy's dinner
Exercise: Dog walk: 12,847 steps

Exercise Win

It's Sunday, my day of rest. But there are no days of rest from dog walking in my new way of living. I know I must go forth, into the wilderness, with my five dogs, and conquer the world. Soon.

Walking is my new rest.

I have work to do, a book to finish by the August 21 deadline, a report to edit for an oil company, books to read and review, but still I fit in exercise, for the good of the dogs and me. I used to walk because I had to; it is a requirement of dog owners, one that is only fair to them and the right thing to do. But it was always painful to pull myself away from the looming stress of deadlines to take a break.

Now, the walk comes first, then the work. Work can wait. Exercise can't. New attitude = new body = health = longer, better life.

August 17, Monday

Weight: 156.7
Ate: 2 Amy's burritos, 2 smoothies, ¼ cup of seeds, ½ avocado
Exercise: Dog walk: 11,139 steps

First Day of School

Year after year, I've watched him go. Always the same thoughts.

"Be okay, son. Be safe. Be kind to him, world."

Then you let him go. Your baby. Your child. Your truest, richest love.

Today he starts his sophomore year of high school.

Only 2 more years after this one to say goodbye to him the first day of school. After that, he will do what most Alaskan 18 year olds do and flee this state to go to college elsewhere, somewhere far away from mom and dad. It will break my heart, maybe break me altogether.

I depend too much on my only son, my only child.

He is my life, really.

Stay safe son, be good, have a good day.

Remember me.

Have a good life.

I'll miss you.

Ah, how hard it is to watch them grow up and away from us, and yet how beautiful too. How precious my life has been to have him in it.

August 18, Tuesday

Weight: 155.4
Ate: 2 Amy's burritos, 1 smoothie, 3 crackers, ½ cup chocolate-covered almonds, 1 cup of soup
Exercise: Dog walk: 10,486 steps

155: Been Here Before...

Three times in the last 15 years since my son was born, I have reached 155 pounds.

It's an incredible weight, so close, 10 pounds close, to victory.

Three times I gained it all back, plus some.

Why?

Why did I work so hard to lose so much, at least 50 pounds each time, just to turn around and go full-throttle into obesity, failure, bingeing, and the depression and shame those things bring me?

Um, because I like chocolate? That's the simple answer.

Um, because I got injured and had to have surgeries? That's the more reasonable answer, but not the entire truth.

The truth is, I got discouraged. I lost my confidence. I came to see myself as a failure. I gave up.

Yep, I just gave up. That's the real reason for the diving back into my eating disorder.

Plateaus killed me, my very spirit, my belief in myself.

What's different this time?

Well, first thing is, I don't care so much about a number, such as 145 or 140. It would be nice…but…155 is nice. Much nicer than 165, or 175, or 210 (January 1 of this year), or even 240, which I was 16 months ago. Sure, I like nice rounded numbers; the idea of losing exactly 100 pounds sounds so awesome, and doable, right down to 140, and victory.

But it might not happen. So what? My body is a machine, a much leaner, stronger, better machine than it was at the beginning of this year. It carries me through steep trails on long walks with my dogs. I care about my body now, and my heart specifically, in an entirely different way than those other diets. Back then, I cared only about how I looked. Now I care about my health, longevity, and abilities to do things physically for as long as I can. That's why I was able to give up Diet Coke, sugar, and smoking along this weight loss journey, something I've never done (successfully) before.

Losing weight, and maintaining weight, as I learned in my little no-diet diet experiment from July 8 through August 12 (when I had a smoothie-only day), does not require a lot of time, physical energy, or strict attention to calories. If I stay vegan and keep up my daily dog walks, I should be good. There's even room in there for the occasional treats, such as a vegan chocolate chip cookie or dark chocolate-covered almonds. In fact, I get a little chocolate in my life every day, through the mocha powder in my coffee and the protein powder in my smoothies.

Life is short, and in my life, I like a little sweetness, especially chocolate-flavored. (Note: I found a new kind of mocha powder that has nutritious plant enzymes in it, or so they say, pictured below.)

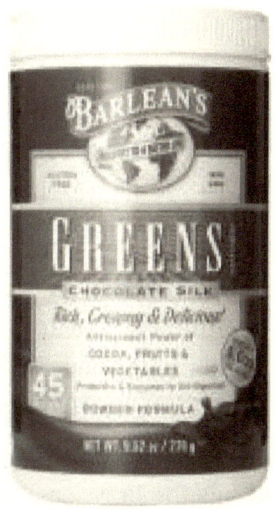

It's working, so who am I to complain?

I can't see anything but success in what I've accomplished so far this year, and what is yet to come. I don't fear the future, as I did before. The only way I can see myself returning to my old habits of bingeing and smoking is in one possible scenario (which I don't even want to consider): if something happened to my son. But then, I don't know if I could even survive such a horror. The least of my worries would be my returning addictions.

August 19, Wednesday

Weight: 155.6
Ate: 1 Amy's burrito, 1 Panini sandwich with veggies and chips, 1 large vegan cookie, 1 smoothie, 1 Amy's spaghetti dinner with 3 crackers, 1 coffee with mocha
Exercise: Dog walk: 16,430 steps

Setting a KOPS Goal and Date

So, October 3 is the TOPS Fall Rally, an annual event wherein all the TOPS groups in the near area come together to celebrate, eat (of course), and…well, I guess that's about all! I usually dread these things, being bored during meetings, but last year the state leader brought her tiny little dog, which made me all happy and content and settled the whole time (I see why people need service dogs for emotional support…it certainly calmed my little ADD brain).

Anyway, the reason I am even bringing up the TOPS Fall Rally is because I've decided to set a goal: to be a KOPS by then. I've never been a KOPS. In my nearly 15 years of being a TOPS member, I've never reached KOPS status. This is the year I will.

The question, of course, is when?

People in the TOPS group are starting to ask if I'm near goal, and I say, "I think I have about 10 pounds of stomach fat to lose." I do, but I don't know that the next 10 pounds will come off my middle. I am sure if I did more weightlifting, I could sculpt it so it would, but I like to do things the lazy, easy way.

In any case, here's my goal:

In six weeks, I will lose 11 pounds, down to 145. I will be at "goal" weight. I will achieve KOPS status.

Calendar	«																					

August 2015

Su	Mo	Tu	We	Th	Fr	Sa
26	27	28	29	30	31	1
2	3	4	5	6	7	8
9	10	11	12	13	14	15
16	17	18	19	20	21	22
23	24	25	26	27	28	29
30	31					

September 2015

Su	Mo	Tu	We	Th	Fr	Sa
30	31	1	2	3	4	5
6	7	8	9	10	11	12
13	14	15	16	17	18	19
20	21	22	23	24	25	26
27	28	29	30			

October 2015

Su	Mo	Tu	We	Th	Fr	Sa
				1	2	3
4	5	6	7	8	9	10
11	12	13	14	15	16	17
18	19	20	21	22	23	24
25	26	27	28	29	30	31

Does this mean I can't lose anymore? No, of course not. I am going to get to where my body is healthiest. But 145 would be – will be – a nice place to be, a good place to strive for. The TOPS "rules" allow for 7 pounds below and 3 pounds above the goal weight to remain a "KOPS":

> *A KOPS goal must be maintained within the following leeway: three pounds above goal weight through seven pounds below goal weight. Example: A member with goal weight of 135 pounds may not exceed 138 pounds or go lower than 128 pounds.*

So what if I lose to 145, then my body decides it is

comfortable at 150? Or (like this would happen) 135?

So much silly things to worry about! If I get and then lose KOPS status, I'm not going to panic about it. I'm just going to be happy to be there. It's been a lot of years, a lot of struggles, a lot of fighting, a lot of hunger and exercise.

It's time to reap the benefits and enjoy.

And then, let the pounds settle where they will. As long as they don't come piling back on. They can stay away for good, as far as I'm concerned!

So, I need to lose 1.7 pounds a week for the next 6 weeks to get to goal. Sounds tough, but I'm tough. Let's do it!

August 20, Thursday

Weight: 157
Ate: 2 smoothies, 2 Amy's meals, 1 avocado, 5 crackers with peanut butter, ¾ cup dark chocolate-covered almonds
Exercise: Dog walk: 16,181 steps

Weight Up

Weight up again, not so much a concern. Just know I have to have a smoothie and soup only day, and increase the exercise a bit.

Just started out for an early morning dog walk, but I didn't get quite 12 minutes in when Chewie told me she couldn't go anymore. She just stopped, stood, and waited for my return. I often look back for her now, as she putters along behind us (then suddenly, she'll hear a squirrel and start running, so I'm confused by how serious this is; is her body breaking down from cancer, has her heavier weight gotten the best of her, is it the thyroid, or is she just being lazy as I often feel?).

Today, she just stood. I was about to make a turn on the trails but looked back, and she was behind me, refusing to move.

"What's the matter, Chewie?" I asked, going back to her, patting her, scratching her now-graying head. "Had enough?"

Yes, she said, by turning toward home.

"Come on, dogs!" I called, and rest came tumbling back, all energy and excitement, confused by our stopping before we'd really gotten into the deep woods, new to them. But they all agreed to be leashed up, and we headed for home.

"Don't worry, I'll walk you all later," I promised, then patted Chewie, "but you can rest at home."

Sigh. Now I have to get the mindset and energy to head out again, instead of getting lost in my computer work. It will be tough, but yesterday I managed to drag myself out for three walks, all Fitbit-inspired, walking all dogs first, then just the puppies, then Miza and Blue on a shorter one.

A Year Ago...

I definitely have more energy and ability now than a year ago.

If I could go back a year from today, I'd see a woman about 225 pounds, in a lot of physical pain, hefting my body on a daily dog walk because that's what dog owners do, but happy when it was over.

I had a lot more work to do, so I sat at the computer longer, perhaps.

If I didn't have a Big Project due, I took a pain pill about 4:00 in the afternoon, when I couldn't bear the agony of my body anymore. I'd crawl in bed with heating pads and dogs and watch TV the rest of the night.

I couldn't see what was just ahead for me:

- In September, going to a writers' conference where I was inspired to finalize and publish my books, winning a prize for best manuscript.
- In October, fostering six puppies that changed my life in so many ways, including showing me that I was capable of much more physical exercise than I thought, as I lost 13 pounds in the 3 weeks they were here.
- Then adopting two of them, Kip and Harper, and being

carried by their love through the winter, busied and tired by their training and the incessant cleanup, happy with their toddler-like adoration.

- Watching my paying jobs dwindle to almost nothing, taking this hard, but keeping busy polishing my books and writing new ones, learning to adjust to a drastically reduced income. Not realizing, entirely, what a blessing it was that I was no longer strapped to the computer 8 to 12 hours a day.

- October through December, inhaling my last holiday candy: mountains of Halloween and Christmas chocolate, not knowing that a year later, I would be vegan and at least six or eight clothes sizes smaller.

- A year ago, I smoked about a pack a day, sometimes struggling to draw them out to two packs every 3 days. When I wasn't smoking, I was missing smoking. I wanted to quit every day of my life, but I couldn't seem to do it. Now, I am a nonsmoker.

Sometimes, perhaps, it's good to think back to a year ago, to see what was accomplished. And then to flash forward. What will my life be like a year from now? Here's some possibilities:

- I don't know that Chewie will be with me anymore. She turns 10 in December, which isn't that old for a dog, but she's not aging well, as some of us don't. I will be, then, down to four dogs, and I won't replace her. The perfect number of dogs is two, I think, but I have done my part to save the world, so here I am, leader of the pack. (Only really, Miza is.)

- I will continue to write and publish; maybe, I'll even find a wider audience for my books.

- I will work hard to improve my relationships with Greg and my son. This is my current project, as I evaluate my ADHD and ways to manage it so that it doesn't affect them in a negative way (my interrupting or being inattentive to them, for example).

- I will, of course, be a KOPS at TOPS. Goal reached, basketball dunked, winner!
- Perhaps I will give up my businesses altogether, replaced only by writing? Tough call when you've spent so many years building businesses from nothing to something.

Who knows what else one year can bring? The last one has been marvelous, I must say.

August 21, Friday

Weight: 157.5
Ate: 2 smoothies, 2 Amy's burritos, ¼ cup of nuts and seeds, 1 cup of soup, 3 crackers
Exercise: Dog walk: 11,017 steps

Panic Eating

The nice part about losing all my files in Dropbox, which means all my files, Wednesday, was I didn't panic eat. Well, in a way I did, but not like the old days, burying my anxiety attack in pounds of sugary chocolate.

When I realized my entire Dropbox folder had been wiped out, both online and on my computer, most probably due to installing the new Windows 10 upgrade on all computers, including my "old" main one (the one that kept crashing in March). Since I still had Dropbox on that computer, I moved all the files off it to a backup drive, deleting them from that folder. What I didn't realize was that online Dropbox considered the "old" computer my main one, somehow, so almost instantly all my files disappeared, including the ones I've been working on with my "new" computer for the last month or so.

In other words, CRAP!

There seemed to be no support number for Dropbox, so finally I filled out every online form I could detailing the problem IN ALL CAPS! WITH EXCLAMATION POINTS!

Then I got in the car and ran away from home.

I'm not really hungry, but I want something; I'm just not sure what. I'm frantic, lost, dazed and confused (ha). So I take my latest book I'm writing (conveniently, on ADHD, another ha!) to Vagabond Blues, order food, and sit down to edit my book.

I eat my vegan cookie. I actually buy a Diet Coke and sip a little of it, not really liking it, but liking the feeling of being "bad" without being bad.

It never even once crossed my mind to have a cigarette, so there's that.

And I didn't finish my food, so there's that.

On the way home, I think to myself, "Well, I guess I'm cured, if the loss of all my files, my history, my work, doesn't drive me to sugar and nicotine." I've come a long way, baby. I – am – cured!

Now I'm back home, piling backup files from a month ago back into the Dropbox folder, knowing I've lost some things, but realizing most of the important files (client's reports; forms I've made) are still resting in my "Sent" Items in Outlook, so they can be recovered. And really, does it matter all that much? Since I survived wiping out one entire 100-page crucial chapter of my dissertation in one swoop, 30 years ago, by saving another chapter over it, I've learned to survive such crises. Life has to go on, anyway, computers or not.

August 22, Saturday

Weight: 157.1
Ate: 2 smoothies, Amy's burrito, 2 smoothies, 1 coffee with mocha, 1 bowl of sweet potato soup plus onion bread, 1 large vegan cookie
Exercise: Dog walk: 19,422 steps

Book Signing #2

Nervous about my book signing today; I don't know why I agree to these things when I really just want to hide out and write books and become famous but no one knows who I really am or where I am....

Marketing. That's what they say it's all about. Especially these days, with so many authors competing in social media for our attention.

Book signings. Why do I do it?

Last time, though, the TOPS and Strong Women ladies showed up in force, supporting me. I don't go to Strong Women anymore, but I can hope some of the TOPS people will come by.

Just don't let me sit there all alone, no books sold, please!

Oh, right, I'm taking Blue. I'll be okay! I'll have a dog to pet. And plenty of (my) books to read!

Later: Well, few people came today. It was a gorgeous Saturday, probably the last summer day of 2015 in Alaska, so I guess most people were doing what I wanted to be doing: hiking in nature. They certainly weren't at the small-town bookstore. Fortunately, a few TOPS friends and my housecleaner came by; some of them felt sorry enough for me to buy a book.

I wondered if my writing career is already over, before it's even really begun. Now that I have time to write and finish my books, does anyone have time to read them?

I take heart in the two nice emails I received from Part 1 of my weight loss journey, some of which I've excerpted below. (Oh, how we writers love to get nice letters and emails from readers! Thank you!)

Letter 1: from D

> I wanted to email you to tell you what an inspiration you are to me! I really enjoy your weight loss journey books and I can't wait for the next volume to come out!

> While I am not a vegan, have no children or "husband," I still relate to you and your writing. You motivate me to keep trying. Very few people I know can relate to "the fat girl got skinny and then gained again" story. Mine was a health issue, but I still feel as if I am judged as if I fell off the thin wagon. It encouraged me when you wrote that this

journey turned from looking good to being healthy for you-
that is exactly what my journey is about this time. I have
also been motivated to do one vegan day a week through
your books. It is a start. I had to read to find out how to do
it. I have chosen the raw vegetable route. Each week I try a
new veggie. My favorite new find is Jicama! I also eat beans
and Quinoa and drink Almond Milk and water. It really is
not bad and I have found that my Vegan day is spilling some
meals over into my normal eating patterns.

I saw the Netflix show you mentioned a few months ago,
along with OMG GMO. Very informative indeed. It saddens
me to see so many young people getting diabetes. I know
from experience that it sucks. I control mine and was only
forced on medication for 3 months over the last 9 years.

You are doing great on your journey and I am rooting
for you daily! Thank you for having the courage to put your
story down for people like me who can use the wit, the
encouragement and the motivation! I read a lot of weight
loss stories and your journey is one of my favorites! Thank
you again and keep up the good work! We will both get to
where we are going...one pound at a time!

Letter 2: from C

I am so happy I stumbled across your books on Kindle. I
really do not remember what prompted me to be interested
enough to download them. I hate all "diet books." In the
past I have spent so much money on every diet book that
came out, and they never stated anything new, and I felt like
the book was written only to make the author as rich as
possible. So for me to become interested enough to even
look into your books....was for certain... divine
intervention. "When the pupil is ready, the teacher
appears."

Within the first few pages, I identified with you in many

ways. I too started the year at 241 pounds and have been steadily losing weight. But unlike you, I am only down to 219 in 7 months. Your book caused me to take a fresh honest look at what I was doing and not doing. First off, I realized that my coffee with Bailey creamer would have to go. Second, I needed to get off my lazy butt and exercise. So now I am doing both….not happy about it yet, but I am doing it. I need to come up with a better plan for exercise. Now I am only walking and deep cleaning my home. I need to join an exercise class or gym so I have a place to go work out when it is 100 degrees.

Anyway, I was sad when I finished your book today, I felt I was losing a friend. So I decided to read your WL Journey all over again.

I could tell you were an ADD'er within the first chapter. Takes one to know one. I just finished a book that says ADD is a gift. The leaders of the world are all ADD'ers, as well as all the creative people and the folks who get things DONE. The winners of the world!!

One more thing, usually when I read a book from Kindle, at the end a page pops up asking for a rating. This did not happen with any of your books? So I was not able to rate your book a 5 star like it deserved. I will go into Amazon and see if I can write a review.

I am very happy for you regarding your weight loss success.

I am so in love with these two women! Thank you for sharing your stories with me and for encouraging me with mine. Together, we will make it! And I loved going back and reading your letters after the book signing went so poorly today; I only sold six books, but hey, that's six books more than I did a year ago!

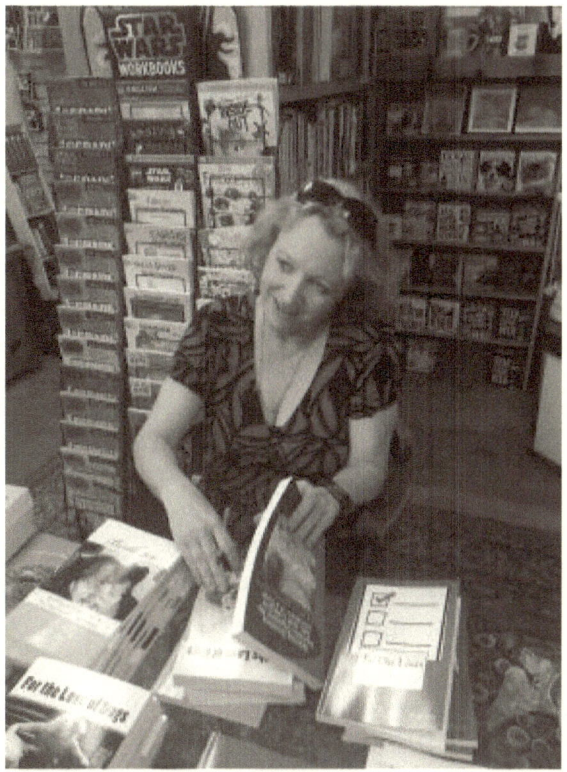

August 23, Sunday

Weight: 157
*Ate: Oatmeal with cinnamon, 2 slices of dry rye toast, 1 order of home
fries, ½ Diet Pepsi, 2 coffees, 2 smoothies, 1 Amy's burrito, 1/3 bag of
kettle corn*
Exercise: Dog walk: 13,455 steps

Best Dog Walk in the World

As I'm researching and writing my latest self-help book, this
one on ADHD, I learn to try to appreciate my moments walking
the dogs more, instead of obsessively worrying about the dogs and
fretting about the trail destruction. I also walk more often alone
(just me and the dogs) again, which is great, because it's my time
to work out issues, think through problems, relax, not have to work
at carrying a conversation or listening attentively to someone else.

Sometimes, I walk all five first, then just the puppies, then the old dogs last (short walk because of Chewie); it doubles my exercise and the second two walks allow me to relax even more since I don't have to constantly be worrying about the puppies being out of my sight in front, potentially getting into trouble, or Chewie falling behind us and getting lost.

Worry worry worry – I am sick of you! So I take steps to conquer you. I will win!

Today, I invited the whole family on the walk, and it was nice. We took the old trail, the one being turned into landfill, which usually upsets me too much to see, but this way I completely relaxed since I wasn't afraid of running into other people and their dogs. It felt so good to be free of worry! God! What a waste of my life worry and anxiety are. How often they have led me to overeating or smoking, now no longer options in my life.

Instead, I journal and walk away my concerns. Nicely done, Jory!

August 24, Monday

Weight: 158.1
Ate: 2 smoothies, 1 cup of split pea soup, ¼ cup of seeds
Exercise: Dog walk: 10,822 steps

Not Enjoying Today

Hungry. Starving. Not how I like to do this. Makes me weak and not wanting to go for a second dog walk. However, I'm up 3 pounds from last week's lowest weight, and the TOPS weigh-in is in the morning, so I thought I'd have a "strict" day of eating, to try to get that scale back down to 155.

There's nothing easy about weight loss, but there is especially nothing easy about those stubborn last 10 pounds. How I hate them! Go away!

(Just kidding; I don't really hate them. They are part of me, just as the last 83 pounds were part of me. They just happen to be an unhealthy part, snuggling around my middle, that I'd like to say goodbye to.)

Fibromyalgia, Fall, and Fat

The last week or so has been one of incredible nasty pain in every joint and just about every muscle…it's what is called fibromyalgia. Little is known about it. I can tell you it's definitely real, and mine seemed to start with the neck injury about 14 years ago. It's like all your pain receptors are turned on but never turn off.

Oddly, it seems to worsen when the weather changes, as I've mentioned. I knew fall was here a few days before the leaves started changing color just by the aching all over, kind of like you have the flu but you don't, and then the tiny sharp jabs of pain elsewhere.

"Do you hurt less now that you've lost weight?" Greg asked.

"No, you'd think so."

"Yes, that's a lot less strain on your knees, for example," he says.

I scowl at him, thinking, *He's getting close to getting in trouble*. But he says nothing else, smartly.

No, no difference. You can't blame fibro pain on fat, my dear Skinny Little Bastard. At least there's that.

In any case, with my pain pills all in my septic tank, there's no chance of me turning to prescription-level drugs for help, which is a good thing. I can take Advil and aspirin if I'm desperate, which I have been the last few days, plus lots of heating pads, a hot blanket, and Ben Gay or Icy Hot rub. Hot baths. Then I try to remember the flaxseed and turmeric pills my brother advised, but which I rarely take (actually, I think he said to sprinkle them on my salads or cook in my food). They are all solutions. They aren't perfect. I know I'll always have this pain. But I live with it, go on, keep walking the dogs, keep working, keep living. What else is one to do? Give up? Never!

Despite the pain telling me fall is here, I feel a general sense of happiness and peace; I love playing Nina Simone's version of "Feeling Good" on YouTube. The lyrics capture my joy when I'm in nature, hiking with the dogs, grateful to still be able to walk:

> *Fish in the sea*
> *You know how I feel*
> *River running free*
> *You know how I feel*
> *Blossom on the tree*
> *You know how I feel*
> *It's a new dawn*
> *It's a new day*
> *It's a new life*
> *For me*
> *And I'm feeling good*

August 25, Tuesday

Weight: 156
Ate: 2 smoothies, 1 veggie burger with fries, 1 Diet Coke, 1 coffee with Greens powder (now using instead of mocha powder)
Exercise: Dog walk: 19,060 steps

TOPS Challenge

Lost 0.4 pound at TOPS today compared to last week. I'll take it! Had to suffer yesterday, a little bit. In other words, I was hungry. And I don't like that feeling. Yuck. Try to avoid it, and most of the time during this journey, I have.

I think about it, and I could eat more vegetables, probably stir fried in water, to eat more plus lose more. I just need to put the effort into actually cooking them.

At the TOPS meeting, I publicized my goal: to reach 145 and KOPS by the October 3 Fall Rally. That would be about 2 pounds a week over the next 5 weeks. It seems impossible, but they were encouraging. The members eagerly agreed to text, email, or call me. Such great supporters! I love them!

August 26, Wednesday

Weight: 156.5
Ate: 2 Amy's frozen meals, 2 smoothies, 1 avocado
Exercise: Dog walk: 13,827 steps

Reshaping and Loose Skin

On the TV reality shows *My 600-lb Life* and *Extreme Weight Loss*, there's a point in the person's journey when she (or he) is often eligible for skin surgery, which sounds incredibly painful and permanently scarring, but of course, the latter show doesn't air any of that, just the happy patient being wheeled away to surgery at 9 months into their journey, and then the successful "reveal" at 12 months. Three months of suffering hidden from the viewers!

Anyway, perhaps you are wondering where I am, having lost 83 pounds in the last 16 months, on top of being age 55 (relevant because, as I noted early in this journey, my neck skin didn't bounce back the last time I lost weight as it always did when I was younger).

So far, so good! No need for skin surgery as far as I can tell. My neck has some sag, for sure, but I was expecting that. I don't think it's as bad as it was last time; perhaps that's because I quit smoking? Or because I still have 10 pounds to lose?

The stomach area still has about 10 pounds to go, and I'm pretty sure it's fat, very little if any extra skin. I do see a few "wrinkles" there, which tells me there might be a tiny bit of a skin issue, but I am sure it is something I can live with.

I don't really see the need (I should say "want") for sagging skin surgery, in any case; perhaps I'd think about it if there were 10 or 20 pounds of skin like on those TV shows, and I was younger and cared how I looked, but I seem to be all right.

August 27, Thursday

Weight: 156.5
Ate: 6 peanut butter crackers, large oatmeal with peanut butter and

cocoa powder, large vegan cookie, 2 Amy's burritos, 1 medium popcorn
Exercise: Dog walk: 11,729 steps

Old Dogs and Jerks

Short dog walk early on gorgeous, quiet trails. All went well except I had to cut the walk in half since Chewie stopped and wouldn't go any more. I love old dogs. They are precious and beautiful. And so what if she can't make it for long walks anymore? So, I adjust and take short ones! And take another one later with the younger dogs.

I guess the reason I'm tirading about this is I dated someone (big mistake, as most of them were!) who, I learned not long before we went our separate ways, got rid of his dog because it couldn't keep up with him anymore. So he dropped it at the pound! Asshole! And he had three beautiful children; he taught them that same lesson….a dog is no good when it can't keep up, so eliminate it.

Ass. And if he hadn't done such an evil thing, I would maybe feel sorry for him, because he missed out on the most beautiful stage of all…the old dog. Sweet, kind, lovely, graying souls of preciousness. They need you, but you have to "read" this. You have to guess on their pain levels, and give medication appropriately. They don't "whine about their conditions," but you'll notice it in the way they slow down, try hard to keep up but can't, want to please you still.

Thank God I am the kind of person who loves old dogs. They are precious, and I am lucky to know them. I'm with you, Chewie. Till the end, beautiful friend.

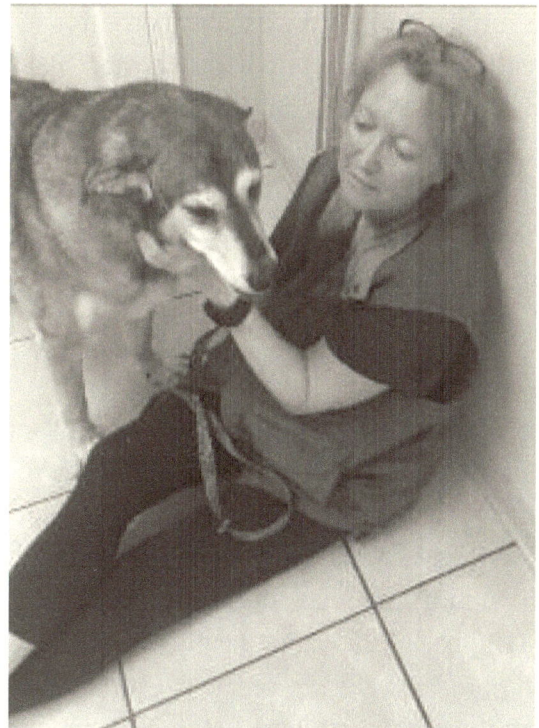

Chewie and me at the vet, again. "There's something wrong," I tell them, but they can't find anything.

August 28, Friday

Weight: 156.1
Ate: 2 smoothies, 1 Amy's burrito, "small" (not really!) bag of nuts at the fair, vegan Boca burger wrap with hummus (at the fair)
Exercise: Dog walk: 11,989 steps

Fair Day #1

And so the Alaska State Fair starts; this is the first year I've prepaid for a season pass, so I can go every day. Of course, the first day cost over $100 in ride and food tickets and games that all players are doomed to lose. But I knew it was perhaps the last time my son would want to "hang" with me at the fair, and even then, not for long. We were both exhausted from trying too hard (I actually tried one ride and the agony on every joint was unbearable), and so I was able to connect with his friend's mother and send the boys off together. I came home for a few hours to wait for his call, covering myself with a heated blanket, putting a heating pad behind my back, slathering my body with Ben Gay, and taking an Advil and turmeric for the fibromyalgia pain. I will get through this, though. I will hold on, keep using natural remedies as much as possible, and have patience and faith that this pain will subside, perhaps as winter storms itself in. Patience, grasshopper!

Fair Food

Speaking of the fair, this is only my second one in my 55 years in which I didn't eat "really bad fattening foods" such as chocolate chip cookies and elephant ears (giant flat donuts smothered in oil, sugar, and cinnamon). I couldn't help but be a little proud walking through the fairgrounds at 156 pounds compared to last year's 226, eating healthy instead of junk.

The food choices were not great. I couldn't find anything to eat that wasn't meat or sugar until I stumbled upon a nut stand. It said hot, sweet, and spicy nuts, but mine ended up being simply some cold Costco mixed nuts poured into a bag, since I said I wanted them "plain." I also ordered the *small* bag, but that was probably a whole cup of nuts…a lot of calories (876, it turns out! Egad!). Boring. Still, proud of me for (1) ordering the small, and (2) not ordering "sweet," which is what I really wanted.

Soon after, I found a booth with a vegan burger, only their bread wasn't vegan so they put it in a wrap. It took me over an hour to eat it, which was impressive. I don't think it's ever taken me more than 5 minutes to eat anything. I just took my time, had a bite here and there, walked around, sat down, had another bite.

I wondered: "Maybe this is how normal, skinny people eat. They take their time." I don't know.

But I'm home now, full, feeling guilty about the nuts, but proud that I avoided cookies, ice cream, elephant ears, pizza, French fries, onion rings, and other fair foods that even as a vegetarian I could slam down my throat. Thank you, Alaska State Fair, for not having many vegan options!

August 29, Saturday

Weight: 158.1
Ate: 2 smoothies (with avocado...what a great pudding texture that gives smoothies!), 1 cup of soup, large bowl of oatmeal with peanut butter and cocoa (Greens powder)
Exercise: Dog walk: 10,051 steps

Falling

What!? Not fair! Up two pounds since yesterday, and I didn't even eat elephant ears or cream puffs! Ha! I'm not really worried. So it will be an "eat-less" kind of day. I tried to "exercise more" but I just took my second dog walk, and both were cut short by Chewie's worsening condition, as she seems to get a little weaker and slower every day. I made another vet appointment while waiting for her during the second walk. It's not the thyroid, it seems; I'm starting to think it's the "Big C" as in fuck cancer; I hate cancer. Cancer killed my father. There are so many things wrong with cancer.

But in any case, no matter what ails her, I will love and spoil this beautiful dog-soul-friend to her end.

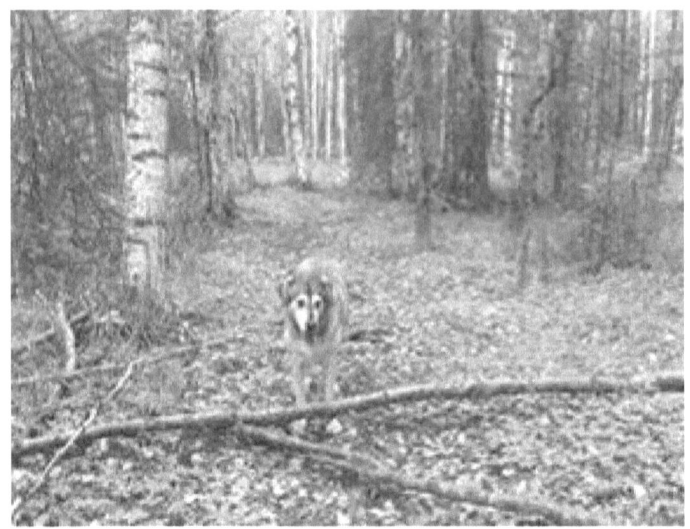

Chewie, finding what was previously a simple obstacle too much to bear.

Fall comes, the temperatures suddenly dipping into the 30s at night the last 2 days, stealing summer from me, throwing leaves on the ground. Fall arrives with winds that toss branches around like the ones blocking Chewie in the photo above.

Fall is here, and it's beautiful, but I hate what this fall symbolizes for me, for my dog. I think this will be a long, dark winter, and my dog will slowly keep fading away from me. Her heart can no longer carry her big body, but oh how she demands to be near me all day. I cannot leave her behind. My walks are shortened, once again, by the love for an aging dog. Every moment left with her is precious. I am lucky to know this, to know her, to know the love of great dogs.

And bad little puppies too.

August 30, Sunday

Weight: 156.1
Ate: 2 smoothies, oatmeal with peanut butter and Greens powder, coffee with Greens powder
Exercise: Dog walk: 12,207 steps

Tips from Healthy Wagers

As I near my HealthyWage.com goal of 153.7, I read some tips from previous winners. Some of them I thought I'd share with you, and I have provided the link to all of them in the Works Cited list.

- Hold your belly button to your backbone hold for as long as you can. Do it every time you think about food. It really works.
- Go for walks rain or shine at least 45 minutes every day.
- Don't eat after 8 p.m.
- Put frozen seedless red grapes in the freezer when you need a snack go for them , they pop in your mouth making you feel very satisfied
- Eat half of what you normally do.
- When craving something unhealthy, chew sugar free gum.
- Patience grasshopper.
- If you run into having a craving for something you think you just have to have, try drinking a full glass of cold water. You might find that it is water your body was craving.
- Count calories with a website like MyFitnessPal and turn up the music and keep moving…you got this!
- Be persistent. You didn't gain the weight overnight and you won't lose it that way. There will be good days and bad days, but no matter what, focus on a goal and stick with it!
- Be 100% committed in your mind! The diet and exercise will follow once you've got your head where it needs to be.
- There is no "quick fix" to losing weight. Learn to eat healthy and celebrate your accomplishments no matter how small they seem to others. Attitude is everything!
- Research, read labels, eat things that you've never heard of or thought you would never eat.
- A little exercise every day, and only comparing yourself

with you.

- There's a ton of ways to lose weight quick, but those same ways also will likely result in putting it back on quick! Focus on healthy, not weight loss. If you can make that switch in your mind, you are golden.
- Pack healthy snacks with you no matter where you go so you don't feel the urge to get something unhealthy while out or at work.
- Completely depriving yourself of favorites leads to cravings. Sometimes just a taste can be very satisfying.
- Write down what you eat and drink. Tracking it really helps.
- Set small goals. That way, the ultimate goal does not seem so far away.
- Do this the healthy way! You need to eat to lose. Starving yourself or eating very little is such an old school way of thinking.
- Clear your environment. Go through your kitchen cabinets and pantry and get rid of all foods that are not consistent with your diet! Then only buy foods that will help you reach your goals for life.
- Believe in yourself and put yourself first. You need to have the belief or a picture of the end result to accomplish your goal and keep you motivated trying to reach it.
- Don't give up during a plateau. Just keep eating right and exercising and eventually it will show again on that scale!
- Do your best and forget the rest. It does not matter how slow you go as long as you keep going!
- Believe in yourself! You can do it! You are worth it!

August 31, Monday

Weight: 156.7
Ate: Smoothies, Amy's burrito, Amy's meal, hummus and crackers
Exercise: Dog walk: 19,111 steps

What I Did Right and Wrong This Month

What I have done right is:

- I stayed with the healthy eating program, especially staying vegan.
- I gave myself a little chocolate treat every day, usually in the form of soy protein powder in my smoothie and Greens chocolate powder in my coffee.
- I made 10,000 steps almost every single day! I even made it over 15,000 some days; this is a huge increase from previous months.
- I started using the Fitbit and challenging my friends. This is what led to the increase in steps.
- I sometimes went on two or even three dog walks instead of just one.
- I kept writing down everything I ate, monitoring it carefully.
- I lost weight! And inches! Slam dunk!
- I attended every TOPS meeting.
- I had a major flare-up of fibromyalgia pain beginning about August 17, which seemed to coincide with the cooler weather, but I kept walking every day even so and avoided pain medications except for an occasional Advil. Instead I used heat and ointments.
- I kept educating myself on nutrition and diets.
- I tried to inspire others, looking outside myself for once, sharing what I've learned if asked.
- I seemed to have dropped another clothes size. My size 10 stretch jeans I ordered are now much too baggy on me. My size XL and L shifts are hanging off me. Nice! Another bag to Goodwill!

What I have done wrong is:

- Of course, I could always exercise more and eat a little less, but these things do not trouble me. The scale is moving closer to goal, slowly, it's true, but it's moving. Overall, I have done well. I am eating "normally," really, as in how I can and probably will eat the rest of my life. I'm good. I'm happy. I'm at peace. And what is amazing is that this is the first time during my journey to wellness that I have said those words: "I'm at peace."

SEPTEMBER

Weight: 155.1 pounds
Exercise: About 12,500 steps a day (dog walks)
Inches: Chest: 42.5 Waist: 35.5 Hips: 41.25
Body Fat %: 27.34 BMI: 26-5/7
Motivation: To win the healthwage.com money! To make KOPS status
at TOPS. To not hurt so much.

September 1, Tuesday

Weight: 155.1
Ate: 1 Amy's burrito, 1 smoothie, dark-chocolate-covered walnuts and
almonds, various smoothie and soup samples, vegan burrito (yucky one)
Exercise: Dog walk: 11,377 steps

Vitamix

I'm at the Alaska State Fair, staring at the Vitamix, sampling the various smoothies and soups. It's a super blender, basically, allowing me to make smoothies of different textures. But it's $450, plus tax, which comes to $462.

That's a lot of dog food.

Do I dare be this selfish?

I dare. Smoothies have changed my life, and my weight, and my health. They are the way I ensure I get fruits and vegetables in my body. I will come back tomorrow, after researching it and checking with friends, making sure it's really worth the money. I will own a Vitamix.

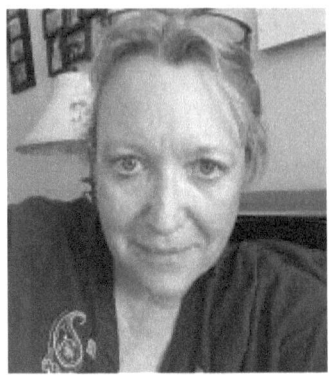

September 2, Wednesday

Weight: 154.7
Ate: 2 smoothies, 2 cups popcorn, 1 Amy's spaghetti dinner, 1 cup of fried potatoes with onions and garlic
Exercise: Dog walk: 14,476 steps

154

What a beautiful number. I stare at the scale, entranced by the "154" on there. It means something special, but as I stand there, nude, I'm not sure what. Victory over so much – so much pain, both physical and mental. So many injuries and surgeries. Pregnancy and childbirth. Raising a child and putting myself last. Thousands upon thousands of hours of work at the computer, desperate to provide a good home and secure college fund for my child. The lowest I've been (by 1 pound) since getting pregnant in 1999, 16 years ago.

Reverse the "5" and the "4" and I'm done. 145. So close. Doable.

I take my moment to reflect, be a little bit proud, then get dressed and get on with the day.

September 3, Thursday

Weight: 156.1
Ate: 3 smoothies, Amy's burrito, coffee with Greens powder
Exercise: Dog walk: 7,943 steps

Baby Time and Vitamixing

Had so much fun yesterday reading to my "baby," Kip, the boy puppy. I'm so in love with him…we are bonded by his desperate need for me, his fear of the unknown, his turning to me with such complete trust and faith for his happiness. Next, I read to a "real" baby, my niece's sweet daughter. They spent the night, and it was wonderful having family around…family who actually talked to me. Nice! (It was also marvelous to see the puppies' complete fascination and gentle kissing of the first human baby they've ever seen…so glad they are kind to children, anyway!)

Enjoying my Vitamix…this morning I made a banana-peanut butter-chocolate soy powder concoction, and later I made the usual, filled with spinach, chocolate, seeds, carrots, and various fruits, but blended to the texture of ice cream. So I made more smoothies than usual. I'm full, happy, and content. I finished a hectic few days of reports and forms, and stayed in bed most of the day (after an early dog walk), reading a book about ADHD.

The rains and wind are hitting Palmer hard today, much more typical of the "fair" weather we expect this time of year than the sunny days I've spent walking around the Alaska State Fair this week. It feels like a serious promise of winter coming, soon. I shiver and snuggle under my covers in anticipation of what is to come, the dogs cloistered around me as if they know too.

You'd think I'd be upset about popping back up to 156 from 154, but I'm good. I know it will all come off, eventually. I'll just keep walking the dogs and eating my smoothies, and we'll see how it goes.

Fortunately, after yesterday's vet appointment, the vet and I agreed to try pain meds for Chewie, so I gave her a Rimadyl this morning, and we were able to take a slightly more robust walk. Maybe it's not cancer that is slowing her down but just pain like I live with, and really, no one should have to live with that. Not if there's a treatment for it. At least, not if you're a dog!

September 4, Friday

Weight: 155.9
Ate: Oatmeal, hash browns, 2 slices of rye toast, 2 giant smoothies
Exercise: Dog walk: 16,590 steps

Sick

Everyone in my family, and just about everyone in Alaska, it seems like, is sick, except me. Yay, plant-based diet! But I feel badly for Greg and Winston, and everyone else, who is suffering from the fall cold virus.

Anyway, yesterday I failed at achieving 10,000 steps for the first time in weeks. I did my dog walk, a nice long one, but then the rest of the day I stayed in bed and read. And read. And read some more. And learned about ADHD. Which I have. And my son seems to have a little jolt of – just the inattentive kind, as in losing things and forgetting to turn in his homework. Another niece will be coming to stay with me soon, tomorrow, it looks like, for several weeks. I'm happy and excited to see her, and also nervous about the idea of having to feed someone who is used to houses filled with food, especially junk food, which I don't buy. We'll see how it goes.

September 5, Saturday

Weight: 155.9
Ate: 2 smoothies, Triscuits with peanut butter; Amy's meal, Amy's burrito
Exercise: Dog walk: 17,143 steps

A Good Day?

The day was good, for me, but I felt like I drove my family mad with my odd humor and interruptions. In fact, we were headed to the fair but never made it. I thought I was funny, but of course, the ADHD education I am embarking on makes me see things from their point of view more. It's tough living with someone with ADHD. I feel a little pity for them. But then my mind thinks of a hundred other things. Distracted, again. Sigh.

September 6, Sunday

Weight: 156.2
Ate: Hummus with veggies, olives, and soft tortillas; smoothie; Triscuits, about 3 cups of kettle corn (popcorn with sugar and salt), ¼ cup sunflower seeds
Exercise: Dog walk: 13,215 steps

Fair-Panic

I'm at the fair, and I know during the hour it takes to drive two miles from my house to the parking lot that it's going to be bad for me. Usually, that drive takes 5 minutes. There's a fall chill to the air, a wetness, a threat. But mostly, it's the people. So many people.

"I feel like I'm in New York City again," I say to my son, panicked, but of course he can't hear me for all the noise of the crowds. I keep losing him, losing Greg, losing my niece. Feeling scared.

I can be alone in the woods with my dogs, out miles from anyone, and happy and at peace (even knowing there are bears, wolves, and moose out there). But crowds of people ruin me. I wonder, "Is anyone here crazed? How many of these people are carrying guns? What if someone goes nuts?"

Several times I walk by smokers, hiding out behind some buildings like criminals, and quickly look away. I want to join them, sneak a cig, breathe it in and let the world disappear. It's the first time I've really missed it in weeks…months? It's been over 16 weeks now since I quit. Over 4 months, according to my Since I Quit app. I take solace in that. I let the craving slide out of me, and I walk away.

I worry too much. But fortunately, after a whole entire hour of waiting for my son and niece to make it to the front of one line for one ride, I convince them to go home. "I miss my dogs. I'm worried about Chewie," I explain, and that is true. But it's also true that I am a person who has never been comfortable in a crowd.

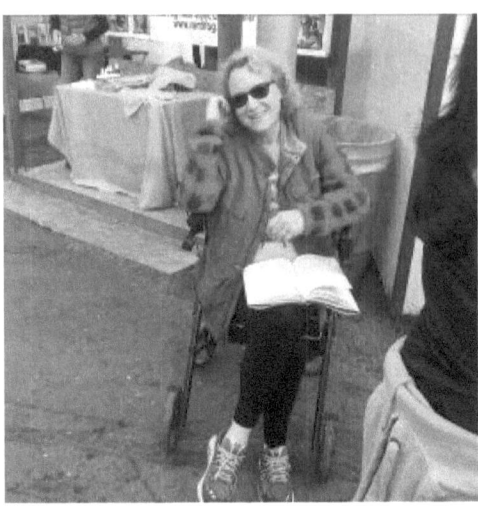

Back at home, I happily make smoothies for everyone, clean house, play with the dogs, watch my niece and son play a board game, then snuggle into my bed and TV, my anxiety pill taking effect, and I feel like I can breathe again.

It's no wonder I spent so much of my life cramming food and cigarette smoke into my body in some odd effort to distract my frightened brain. I forgot to try deep breathing. It would have helped. Fortunately, I brought my godmother's walker and a book to the fair, so even in the midst of crowds, I could find some solace, some peace, sitting and reading, letting the world tumble around me. I tried to remind myself that just this morning, when I drove to Anchorage to get my niece, I stopped by a store and bought myself size 10 jeans, size L leggings, and a size M shirt and coat.

"You bought clothes that fit!" Greg marveled. I took this as the compliment it was intended to be, proud of what I've pulled off. A year ago, at this same fair, I was eating elephant ears and pizza and funnel cakes like everyone else, waddling by the exhibits, triple-chinned but still starving, deep inside, for something, but I didn't know what.

Love, that's what I wanted, after all. I was about to get it, big time, from six little puppies, born wild in Alaska, frightened and needy, missing their mom they'd been pulled from, giving their trust and affection to me. That's when the weight loss seriously began. When I had the love of puppies in my life.

Smoothies?

Today, for the first time since starting my weight-loss journey exactly 9 months ago, I was sick of smoothies. I figured this day would come; I'm surprised it took so long, and ruefully wished it had come a week earlier, before I spent half last month's income on a Vitamix.

Oh well.

So I put the remains of my spinach-carrot-fruit-protein powder-pumpkin seed concoction in the fridge and instead cooked up the giant $5 zucchini I bought at the fair. Turns out it took two of my largest frying pans, plus a pizza tray to bake the rest. Then I put too much soy sauce in the frying pans, so I added in my entire bag of frozen vegetables, plus a box of wild rice I had in the cupboard for probably a decade.

There, done. A nice bowl of rice and veggies. Yum. I'm off to finish it.

The truth is, I'm enjoying another day of reading, but I'm also worried, as my son is spending the day at the fair with my niece. "I don't wanna go," he whispers to me over the phone this morning. "Just go," I say, exasperated with him and with my puppies, who are that moment trying to pull me off my feet as I leash-walk them on the busy-with-weekenders trails. Now, some 6 hours later, he's still at the fair. I'm hoping he comes home tired and happy, like the puppies are after a leash-free walk.

September 7, Monday

Weight: 156.2
Ate: Smoothie, 1 small bag of popcorn, olives, Amy's frozen meal, soup;

fruit, oatmeal, ½ cup seeds
Exercise: Dog walk: 12,514 steps

Labor Day

Labor Day. Makes me think of how much I have overworked most of my life, since I was about 12, honestly.

Labor Day. It makes me think of how much my work has dwindled over the last 3 years, but how, slowly, especially over the last year, I let that go, didn't seek more, quieted, breathed, calmed. And lost weight. And quit smoking. And perhaps will live to see more Labor Days because I improved my health.

I wanted to give myself a firm little pep talk, telling myself this "156" number is ridiculous: "Didn't you make it down to 154 just last week?" But I don't feel like picking on myself. I think of how, yesterday, I picked up my niece and bought pizza for the family plus watched everyone consume incredible-looking fair food later, and I didn't imbibe. I stuck with a couple cups of kettle corn, which is bad enough.

Labor Day. How I love that I can relax, read books, walk my dogs, and work from home. I am blessed. I am happy. (Now if only the stock market would quit tumbling so I can relax about all the money I've worked so hard to earn and gave to my investment guy, just so that I can take time off to write.)

How a Day Can Turn Wrong So Fast

This puppy is a problem. A serious problem.

I suppose you all knew that already, reading along on my happy little walks, once in a while (really just once?) interrupted by Kip's chaotic sudden aggression toward another dog, zip in and out, done, but trauma all around?

Happy walk this morning on the trails; almost back, calling up to Greg at the point where we need to leash the puppies; he barks back in anger at me, "I know!" but I am distracted, talking with my niece, walking slowly behind with old Chewie, and then it happens.

A family, with dogs, everyone off leash; my pack piles into theirs, and Kip is the cause of everything bad, jumping from one dog to another, landing on a little dog, which Greg says he threw in the air. I'm there now, leashing Kip, who's left the chaos as quickly as he entered, coming proudly to me to tell me about his hard work, but the man is screaming, "Which dog was it? I will kill him!" and I truly think he will. The man is calling Greg – who really has nothing to do with any of this except he puts up with me, the person who rescued five dogs – every cuss word in the world. (My son got to hear some words he never heard before.)

The little dog looks okay to me, but the man's fury frightens me away, just as Kip's has frightened all of us, and so we hurry home, ashamed and worried. What do I do? I head to a pet store with Kip, buying the first muzzle in all my years with dogs, plus a harness to grab him by. Kip stands, confused, frightened, trying to remove the muzzle, but mostly looking at me, questioning, "Okay?"

"Yes, it's okay," I assure him, amazed in all this still how I am the person he turns to for all answers; I am the one he trusts; I am the one he loves. I walk him around the store and pick up a tennis ball for him. Of course he can't hold it with his muzzle on, but he immediately perks up in happiness, his body relaxes, he eases into me. The muzzle is forgotten and his focus is only on the ball.

Why little Kip, little boy? Where does this strange aggression come from? It seems to be all wrapped in fear…terror of other dogs, and yet you get along nicely with mine, did fine in puppy class, trust me on the leash. But still, I remember you as a tiny puppy about one year ago, petrified of me and everyone else, trying to hide while your brothers and sisters snuggled into me excitedly and explored the new world of my house and yard with enthusiasm. No, you were different. Bigger than them, you shook in fear at every sound, light, noise. I made you my special project.

I will teach him to trust, I thought, and so I did. Watching your fear of me shift to curiosity, acceptance, and finally glee over the next few weeks was amazing. I of course was doomed to adopt you, although I told everyone no way am I getting another dog.

I think curiously about Kip and his dog-brain now. It's an odd one, different than any I've known before. Of course, all dogs, like humans, are unique, but usually there are similarities, things that make sense. For example, when Mr. Angry Man was screaming this morning, four of my dogs were still, staring at him, watching, trying to understand. One just paced, his eyes dancing around his head, coming to me, oblivious to what was being said or what he had done. Something in those unsteady eyes…something odd, and beautiful too. Something that doesn't make sense; something unique; something special. If only I can teach him not to be reactive, he will be one incredible dog for my next decade or so!

Ah, my Kip, why must you be trouble to me? I am well into my middle age; things are supposed to be gentling down now, getting easier at last. Life is not supposed to be so hard. You are making it both joyful and sorrowful at the same time, Kip, with your intense affection for me and your odd outbursts.

Perhaps, forever, you can only be on a leash when I walk the woods; forever, you can only be muzzled when out. Perhaps, forever, you will be afraid; I can never trust you again, like an abusive boyfriend.

"We should just drop him off there," Greg mumbles, knowing it's not possible of course, as he drives past animal control. For the first time in my 55 years, I might understand why people do that, just a little, although of course I wouldn't consider it.

I hope, of course, that animal control doesn't show up and take Kip, but they might. I have little doubt that the rightfully angry man will file a complaint, and then if they figure out who we are (which won't be hard, because who else has five dogs PLUS did the right thing and applied for the kennel license, and even went much farther by including pictures and descriptions of every dog in case one ever got lost?). Shit. So my mind wanders to Kip going to animal control jail, then murdered by them, me killing myself in sorrow, Greg getting sued by Angry Man and losing everything, my son homeless and penniless and motherless and Kipless.

I force these thoughts away, replace them with images of never having to worry about Kip again now that he has his super muzzle. Of course, as soon as I got him back to the car, I yanked it off and gave him his ball, and now, half an hour later, he plays happily with it and his sister behind me while I type, panting in total joy, rolling and lolling like the puppy he still seems to be, unaware that he is a dangerous idiot dog who has scared the hell out of two entire families today.

At least he didn't drive me to food. Except for free popcorn at the pet store. I did do that. I blame him entirely.

September 8, Tuesday

Weight: 154.8
Ate: Coffee with Greens powder, large vegan burrito and chips with tons of veggies and rice, oatmeal with peanut butter and cocoa
Exercise: Dog walk: 13,622 steps

First dog walk ever with a muzzled dog, the puppy-of-trouble, Kip. I got a large basket muzzle so I can give him treats and he can pant. He seemed to adjust okay. Puppies are pretty adaptable.

It is nighttime now, but it's been a long hard day, started with an early rush to the vet with Chewie, whom I had to leave there while they ran tests. Her mouth and nose started pooling blood. Her tongue and gums went white. I'm losing her; I'm losing her; I knew it. But I still had to pay the $700 to get the confirmation.

"That can't be right," the vet says, after seeing her blood work. "There are no platelets." She takes Chewie in, saying she'll run another more comprehensive test. Plus x-rays and ultrasound.

I already know, but I must try anyway.

I think Chewie's fate was sealed some 8 years ago (March

2007, to be exact), when she munched her way through a drawer of China-made and China-poisoned Old Roy's peanut butter dog biscuits I'd bought at Walmart. Extreme vomiting, emergency vet visits, IVs for days. The "recall" promised pet owners reimbursement for vet bills, but of course this was a lie, at least for me and Chewie. I was lucky she survived it. But I can't help think it's what is killing her now, years away, while her sister still dances happily through the woods and house, puppyish still at just 3 months shy of 10 years old.

Later, I pick her up. "Well, you called it," the vet said quietly. "You know your dog." She seemed to admire how I could tell, all summer, bringing her in, saying, "My dog is dying. There is something seriously wrong," even though all the blood tests showed her as normal, and her heart beat soundly, her tail wagged, her appetite was unchanged. Suddenly, she has no platelets left. Her immune system is under attack. There is really no chance of survival. The vet pumps tons of steroids in her, and at this news, looking at my dog collapsed on the vet clinic floor (I've brought a blanket in for her, so at least she's comfortable), I know I won't have a brief month or two of miracle cure like with Buddy, where he felt better on steroids, although crazed with hunger.

So, I bring my old friend home to die. I love her. I appreciate what we've had together. I am in for hard days.

Food is suddenly the last thing on my mind. And hers. Two species always bonded in so many ways, including by our love of eating, lie together, waiting. And me? I reflect on 9 years and 9 months of one good amazing kind friend.

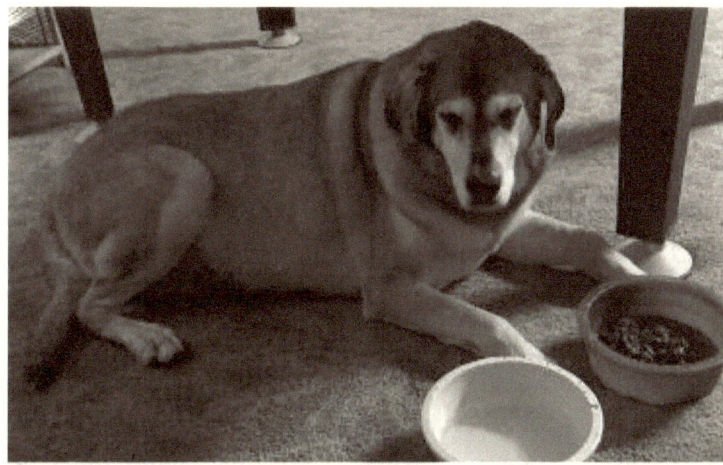

Chewie today. She is swelling up, her blood unable to clot, especially in her neck where the vet drew blood. You can see how swollen her neck is getting, filling with blood.

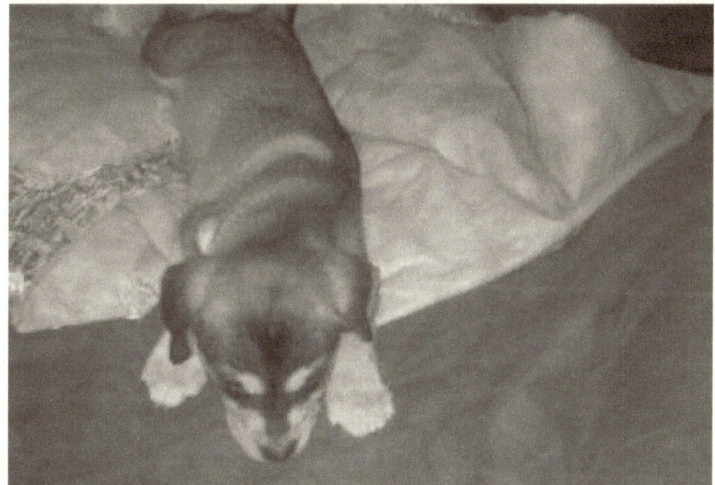

Chewie as a puppy, 9 years and 9 months ago.

September 9, Wednesday

Weight: 155
Ate: Smoothie, spaghetti, 2 slices of toast with avocado and salsa, chocolate walnut vegan cookie, avocado with peanut butter and banana and cocoa smoothie
Exercise: Dog walk: 19,389 steps

Love, God, and My Dog Chewie

Chewie's fading away, unable to eat or drink today, wanting to spend her last hours outside on the grass in the sun. I have had some special time with her today, and I like how the sun reminded me of God in our "selfie" (below). I know she's a lucky dog, as I have told many others during this "time." I have seen many things over my years volunteering, including puppies and young dogs who never had a chance at life because there are too many, and old dogs abandoned instead of loved at the end. Chewie and I have slept 3,600 nights together and taken over 3,000 walks together on various trails and parks in Alaska. She has swam in dozens of rivers, lakes, and ponds. She has never gone a day without food or a night without a toy. I have never gone a moment without her love. I will miss her, but I also feel so happy and blessed to have known her.

September 10, Thursday

Weight: 155.4
Ate: Rice and veggies bowl, coffee with Greens powder, oatmeal with peanut butter and chocolate, spaghetti with bread, chocolate almonds
Exercise: Dog walk: 10,389 steps

The Last Walk

I ate well yesterday, surprisingly, as I didn't think I'd eat at all, based on my mood, watching my dog fade. I took incredible joy in the two times she ate a little (canned cat food), both times allowing me to get the steroid pills into her.

In the morning, the other four dogs tumbled energetically past her, ready for their walk, and she struggled up and after us, slowly. I gave the leashes to Greg and my niece, and I stayed with Chewie, walking her behind the barn, letting her sniff the air casually, then she turned around. Well, we had this then, I thought, our own special little walk together. Later, when she was settled back home, I went and caught up with the others. So I got in my "steps" for the day, but most of them going up and downstairs from Chewie to my space upstairs, which, for the first time in her life, she didn't try to make.

Ah me. It is hard losing a dog.

September 11, Friday

Weight: 155.8
Ate: Oatmeal with cinnamon, 1.5 pieces of dry rye toast, 1 order of hash browns, 1 Diet Coke, 1 coffee with Greens powder, Amy's burritos, smoothie, hummus with crackers
Exercise: Dog walk: 8,884 steps

A Soul Leaves Me

You would think it would get easier, this losing a dog, after so many years of old dogs passing away and leaving me behind. The thing is, the only real flaw you know dogs have is that they have such short life spans compared to ours. So yesterday, as she vomits up blood, can't walk, leans on me to keep from falling into the pond (where I dreamt her body was lying the night before), I know I have to take her to the vet and end this suffering. Still polite, even as she's weakened, can't eat or drink, and can't seem to move, she somehow managed to make it all the way up the stairs last night to the doggie door, while I slept, to go outside and vomit piles of blood. Sweet, considerate, suffering girl.

I arrive at the vet's, ask them to come out to the car to do it, and I hold her and say goodbye while they put the first shot in, the one that helps her into deep sleep. I try not to let her know I am crying, to talk gently and softly as I say goodbye, to pretend for her that I'll be all right. Then I let go and back away while the final shot is given, the one that stops the heart.

Later, I'm trying to help Greg dig the hole, but I stumble away, to the car. I drive to the store, the place where I go for life's traumas. No, I didn't get cigarettes, or cookies, or ice cream. I got a Diet Coke and vegan dark chocolate covered almonds.

Fuck diets, I think, but still I managed to stay with it, stay vegan, not buy cigarettes. Still, in my grief, through my mind, spun

9 years and 9 months of life together, not enough time, but still all precious. As well as thousands of walks, there were surely over a thousand car rides, always a lovely time for her, a precious time. As I'm driving, I look up at the sky and have to pull over in amazement. A giant dog cloud, surely in the shape of a younger, happier, laughing Chewie, is galloping over Pioneer Peak. By the time I have the phone out to take a picture, the cloud is wisping away, changing, moving on. Like she did.

No doubt at all she was my best-behaved dog, except for snapping Harper Lee when the puppy came too close to her bowl (just once was enough) and the desire to break into the garbage container seeking cans. She was always hungry, always on a diet – to no avail – the last few years, as her weight continued to creep up for no apparent reason while her sister stayed slim.

Today is a day of remembrance for other reasons that have nothing to do with some middle-aged lady's dead old dog in Alaska, and so I record the 9/11 specials, planning to crawl into bed to watch them and cry for the people who died so unfairly, and cry for the dog who lived a good life, died a fairly gentle death, and who will be missed by me the rest of my life. Goodbye, dear Chewie, my friend. This morning, I walk four dogs, down by the river, Kip in his muzzle, Miza in a bark collar, and think of the one who was always well behaved, never a problem, and wish she was here, running in the sand, licking the salty driftwood, grinning at me gratefully when I walked up to her.

September 12, Saturday

Weight: 155
Ate: Smoothie, hummus with crackers, carrots, Amy's burrito, chili with tortilla wrap
Exercise: 7,577 steps

In Bed

Yesterday I deleted all social media from my phone and computer (thinking someone would notice, but they didn't). I silenced my phone (as if anyone ever calls; they don't). I took my niece to Anchorage in the morning so she can hang out with the happy, busy family of my brother while I steep myself in the quietude of mourning.

Today, I took no dog walk. The four dogs were tolerant of this; they seemed fine to hang out with me in bed all day (although I felt reams of guilt). Lots of scratching and chew toys, plus special hugs for Blue, whose sister will never run beside her again.

I read and watched one documentary, *Oxyana*, which is about prescription drug abuse in Oceana, West Virginia. How tragic to see the waste of young lives. "Read, son!" I think, as I watch it, realizing not one of these trailers seemed to have a book in it, and wondering if diving into literature would have given them enough of a high to avoid shooting up Oxycontin). I'm so grateful, with my addictive tendencies (sugar, cigarettes) that I didn't get addicted to pain pills, even though I had a cabinet filled with them, and a body that shoots pain signals to my brain every minute, day and night. Proud of myself for dumping those pills in the septic tank.

I am a reader, and it is what saves me from my despair. I end the day of mourning with gratitude for my good life, my kind parents, my education, my son, my interests, and for the joy of knowing pure love from my dogs, even if they do die after a mere decade or so of life and break my heart. It is worth it, I think, fallings asleep with Kip in my arms, snuggling me, and Harper wrapped around my legs, sighing.

September 13, Sunday

Weight: 154.4
Ate: Smoothie, soup, oatmeal with peanut butter and chocolate, coffee with Greens powder, carrots with hummus, Amy's burrito
Exercise: Dog walk: 5,262 steps on Fitbit (plus 4,790 dog walk; forgot Fitbit)

September Morn

It's morning. I got up early, dragging myself on a dog walk before 8 a.m. to try to avoid the morning crowds and the potential headache from the now-muzzled (but still I'm concerned) Kip. It's cool, 36 degrees, the first real snow of fall thick on the mountaintops that surround me.

The walk goes well; I start to panic as we head toward home and leash them all…just four now. Feel a sense of gladness that the walk is over. Instead of a joyful part of my day, it has become a chore that must be done early, before the crowds line the trail, or just one person with a dog. Greg is along too, of course. This is the way my walks have to be now that I have "bad puppies." No longer are my walks quiet and peaceful, but instead, I am filled with anxiety for how the puppies will behave if we encounter another dog. No longer can I walk alone with my pack. It is not bears, moose, wolves, or coyotes I fear, but people with dogs. I suppose I could just take Blue out, alone, sometime, and get that same feeling of peace in the woods I used to have. But even she acted up once last week, snapping at a sweet, old retriever that was passing us. What is happening to my dogs? *Et tu, Blue?* Who has been sweet to all dogs for over 9.5 years? *Et tu?*

Perhaps I will have to learn to find peace at the gym. What an odd, impossible concept. I can't imagine being in a den of sweat, locked in with other people, especially the perky but always slightly nasty little employee girls, no dogs, no trees…how can that calm me?

On the other hand, I know my health is important to me now, not just how my body *looks*, but how it *functions*. I started today's walk by falling, hard, so fiercely that my left leg (the one with the two knee surgeries already) was folded completely under me. I had slipped on Kip's leash as he ran by before we got out of the yard. I pulled myself up, pleased. I had not torn or broken anything, unlike previous falls. I did not require surgery. This body did not betray me. Yes, it hurts, but it always hurts. The point is, I can fall without severe consequences. I can fall again. I am healing.

0.8 Pounds to Go

I didn't take joy in the number on the scale this morning as I should have, as I was fretting about the walk, anxious, and missing Chewie. But now I can look back and think, well, I'm less than a pound away from meeting my HealthyWage.com goal and money. I am one day away, if I do it right. At 153.6 pounds, I will win the prize: $1,324. (Of course, I probably can't officially weigh in and get my $ till mid-October, but I'm good with that. What's wrong with hitting it a month early? By mid-October, I'll be in the 140s, and to my TOPS final goal.)

September 14, Monday

Weight: 152.6
Ate: Smoothie, Amy's burrito, ¼ cup of seeds, large bowl of oatmeal with peanut butter and chocolate, coffee with Greens powder
Exercise: Dog walk and treadmilling: 9,166 steps

HealthyWage Goal Earned (but not counted)

Went right through the healthywage.com goal of 153.6, skipping from 153.6 at 5 a.m. to 152.6 at 8 a.m. This should be a day of joy, but of course, I am still in the throws of grief for Chewie. Still, I made it and sent an email to healthywage. I have a feeling they are going to make me wait until my "weigh-out range" of October 10-24 to submit the video and whatever paperwork is required. But on a normal day, this would feel great.

Later: Heard back. Yes, I have to wait till October 10:

> *Congratulations on your weight loss. We do not accept early weigh ins. Your weight out has to be done between the 10th and the 24th of next month. This will give you time to maintain your new weight, which will help you in the long run. The best way to not trigger a second weigh in is to upload a video.*

I'm not sure I appreciate the "this will give you time to…" whatever tone, the typical lecturing tone toward fat people. If I'd reached my goal October 10, I would get my money without the lecture. But oh well, I'll wait. I have no worries that I'll gain any back in the next month. (And how nice it is not to have that worry.)

Social Square

I've disappeared from all social accounts such as Facebook, Fitbit contests, and Twitter (the latter, I rarely used) since Chewie died. You'd think someone would notice or care. I peek at Facebook several times a day to see if I'm missed.

Turns out I'm not.

I need to get "real" friends instead of virtual ones.

Work

A week of no work awaits me. I guess that's a good thing. I will walk dogs, read books, write books. But it also saddens me a little. I miss the money, sure, but more I miss the throwing myself into huge projects, getting lost in them, turning mediocre documents into great ones. I miss the pleasure of the praise from clients.

But even more, I like the freedom and "living the dream" life I have now. I have shifted careers over the last year. Friday will mark one year since I went to a writers' conference that changed everything, helped me to "let go" of my technical editing career and shift to a new one, although actually my first and longest career: writing. I knew in fourth grade when a check arrived from Archie Comic Books telling me my letter on dinosaurs was to be published that this was the career for me. In the years and careers since, I have published hundreds of stories, articles, editorials, and poems but never worked at it full time.

Now I give myself this gift, for the last part of my life. Perhaps I will find financial as well as personal success at it, but either way, I'm doing it, because it's in my fingers, my soul, my being…to write, to share, to publish. To reach an audience.

Today, as I walked the trails, I had a different attitude than usual. I appreciated them in their fall glory of sharp odors and colors. Then I accepted that they will be gone, forever, and I will be okay with that. What else can I be? Angry and hateful and resentful forever? No, I let them go, into landfill, sadly, but accepting. So too, I let go of my last and wonderful careers: document designer and technical editor. They served me well, paid me exceedingly well, and allowed me to work at home for most of my child's life so far. For all that, I am grateful. But it's over now. A new career awaits.

September 15, Tuesday

Weight: 153.8
Ate: 2 smoothies, coffee with Greens powder, bowl of chips with salsa and veggies, oatmeal with peanut butter and chocolate, Amy's frozen breakfast meal
Exercise: Dog walk: 10,401 steps
Inches: Chest: 42.5 Waist: 35 Hips: 40.5
Body Fat %: 27.18; BMI: 26-1/3

Body Fat Percentage

Weight loss stats are looking good. As well as losing 57 pounds this year, I've lost over 10 inches from my waist and almost 10 from my hips. My BMI has dropped 9-5/7 points, still in the overweight range at 26-1/3, but nearing the "normal" healthy BMI range of 19.1-25.8. A lot of dog walks I took, and a lot of chocolate I did *not* eat. Oh yes, and I've now been a nonsmoker for 17 weeks and 5 days!

The body fat percentage is 27.18. I was concerned about this, mostly because even though I take a long dog walk every day, I don't really do much by way of exercise. I tend to "meander" more than walk, and I don't lift weights since quitting the Strong Women classes although I keep meaning to add that to my weekly to-do list. But it looks like I'm doing well, per the "Ideal Body Fat

Percentage Chart":

ACE Body Fat % Chart		
Description	Women	Men
Essential fat	10-13%	2-5%
Athletes	14-20%	6-13%
Fitness	21-24%	14-17%
Average	25-31%	18-24%
Obese	32%+	25%+

Source: Builtlean.com

I'm doing well; I'm good. I'm so close (and yet so far, as those last 10 pounds feel like) to being done. My body is starting to feel almost "right"; it is nearing the sleekness I used to know and love back before I had a baby (and no, I don't blame him; I love and worship him!). It's exciting, really, the thought of losing that last pouch of fat on my belly and back. I welcome it.

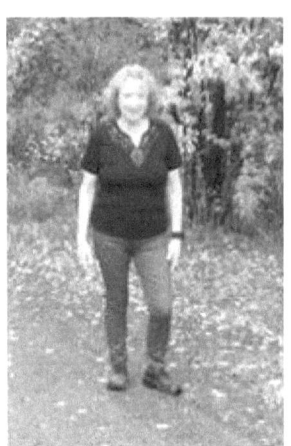 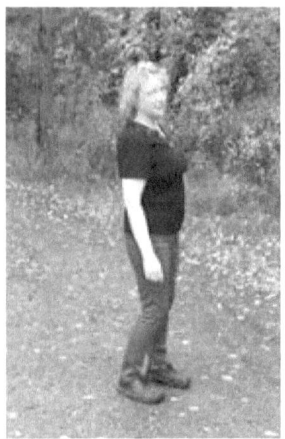

TOPS Queen?

Today our TOPS group had a visitor, the area captain. "You must be close to goal," she said to me, and I said, "Well...." Noncommittally. I don't really know what my goal is. It's not exact a number, but a place, a state, where my body feels right and good and stops losing. That might be now, or it might be 10 pounds from now, or even more. So that's what I meant by "Well…."

Later, as she's talking, she mentions something about "in case the state queen is from our area." I feel eyes on me. It's a good feeling.

For the first time, I think, maybe being state queen is something I actually want. Not only a couple free nights in a hotel for the state meeting but a free trip to Orlando next summer (although I wish it was in winter!). Maybe I want something more. Maybe I deserve to have a crown on my head and the word "congratulations" tossed at me. Maybe what mortified me before – the thought of being the center of attention because of my weight – would actually be a wonderful thing. Maybe I deserve some praise for the battle I've fought and am coming so close to winning.

Maybe.

September 16, Wednesday

Weight: 154.2
Ate: 2 smoothies, Amy's meal, hummus and veggies
Exercise: Dog walk: 11,319 steps

Fat Shaming Video

Okay YouTube, I'm not impressed that you removed Nicole Arbour's so-called "fat shaming" video, especially when my own niece, a mere child, watched the horrible ISIS murders on your website. Really? You're going to censor some comedian who criticizes fat people?

Look, I understand, fat shaming is mean and wrong and all that.

But we also have freedom of speech in this country.

And I don't need you to protect me from people's fat jokes. I can take it. I'm tough. Tough enough to bounce up and down the scale of obesity several times.

I do a search and find the video that the Internet and news

anchors and writers desperate for a subject are busy slamming.

Anyway, the video is back on YouTube on various reposts, fortunately. I didn't think it was so bad. "Fat shaming is not a thing," she argues. "Big boned isn't a thing."

> *"They forgot to tell you that plus sized means plus heart disease. Plus knee problems. Plus diabetes. Plus your family and friends crying because they lost you too soon because you needed to have a Coke plus fries."*

Good one. But Erica Watson doesn't think so. In her response essay on Ebony.com, she writes:

> There is nothing wrong with being plus sized. The body acceptance movement is a REAL THING. There are plus positive women who are truly making an impact and social media is just one of their tools. From events like The Fuller Woman Expo, Curvy Con and Full Figured Fashion Week, to social media campaign's such as Lane Bryant's #PlusisEqual, Tess Muenster's #effyourbeautystandards and Wear Your Voice Mag's #DropTheTowel are providing a platform to show that body confidence and loving our body are themes that all women need to embrace. I thank God that there are magazines like Plus Model Magazine, Slink and Daily Venus Diva that truly speak to showing the diversity in beauty. By embracing this movement, all women, no matter what size can feel good about loving themselves and living a fulfilled life!

Whatever. I'm just presenting the news here, not getting in a fight. I'm just sticking with my "simple" little diet and daily walking program, living my live, slowly losing the pounds. Oh yes, make that 87 pounds in the last 17 months, or 68 weeks. Averaging 1.2 pounds a week. The right way to do it, I'm told, a comfortable way, an anyone-can-do-this kind of way. A way that is so slow it becomes a new lifestyle.

I'm not shaming fat people. I love fat people. I was one. I still have at least 10 pounds of fat resting on my stomach and back. The only time I feel like "shaming" fat people is when their children are fat. I know it's impossible to control everything your child eats or doesn't eat, though. I get this. My child is more food-picky than anyone, including me.

But I have noticed how much more he exercises now that his dad and I have made it a daily habit for ourselves and how much less he eats since I don't buy junk food anymore. Before, if I bought him a soda, he'd drink it. If I bought him Cheetos or potato chips, he'd eat them. So guess what? I don't buy them. He just ate a snack of fresh grapes because that's what was available. Win.

I get a little upset when I see fat children because often the house and cupboards are stuffed full of crappy food. I know. I grew up that way too. Sugar cereal for breakfast, plus cookies and snack cakes when I got home. Ice cream galore.

What if there had been carrots on the counter instead of homemade chocolate chip cookies? Would I have had to struggle with fat for all the 50+ years? (Do I sound like I'm blaming my mother? I don't mean to. I loved her, and she is long gone and cannot defend herself. On the other hand, what I mean is, they are children. They don't buy the food that is placed before them. We are their role models and their suppliers.)

September 17, Thursday

Weight: 154.4
Ate: Smoothie, oatmeal with peanut butter and chocolate, Amy's frozen meal, hummus with carrots
Exercise: Dog walk: 6,528 steps

Snow

Each morning since Chewie died, I peak out my back deck at the mountains and see the snow. It is easing down a little more each day, coming for me, for all of us down here. It will be a long, brutal winter. I only take solace in the idea of spring some 7 months away. Winter will come and punish me, but spring will come too.

Punish me? Odd choice of words. What have I to be punished for?

After a loved one dies, there's that sweeping sense of guilt; I could have, should have. Of course, I did everything right with her. I took her to the vet, lots. I tried to save her from her suffering, her end.

But what I have to be ashamed of is the puppies. Bringing them into our home, turning my full attention from Chewie to them, overwhelming them with my love. Here's the real shame: choosing them over her.

"Don't you understand, Chewie? This is my nature. This is why I saved you too," I'd try to explain, as she stared at me hugging Kip and Harper, sad and angry. Maybe not angry. Maybe just hurt.

Did she die of a broken heart?

And I am left with the hell that is Kip, afraid of what he will do to other dogs, afraid of the lawsuits and screams. Yet, when we aren't on the trails, but are safe at home, he is fine, snuggling into my arms and staying there, just like he's been doing for the last 11 months. Only now when he does it, Chewie isn't looking at me with eyes of jealousy anymore.

I miss you, my dear dog. And I'm very sorry that your last year was spent watching me fall in love with two black puppies. I wish I could tell you that I never stopped loving you, too. But you aren't here to convince.

French Fries and Burger King

So I'm standing in Burger King, after a short dog walk, planning to order a veggie burger with fries and a Diet Coke. These are all things I rarely eat...maybe once a month since starting this diet. I know I've been brought here by the McDonald's French fry commercial I tried to forward through last night on TV. "Crap. Now I want fries," I thought. Brainwashed to crave them. I pulled into Burger King without much thought. Just as the TV and magazine ads for smoking helped turn me into a nicotine addict, so the fat-foods (yes, I meant "fat" not "fast") commercials turn us into consumers of foods that are rotten for our body.

The smell when I walked in was overpowering. Chicken. As in dead, cooked chicken. It made me sick.

Fortunately, while I waited for the elderly gentleman to make up his mind, staring at the chicken "fries" pictures, I thought about the chickens being sliced and cooked for Burger King foods. I thought mostly about their miserable factory-farmed lives and the terror of their slaughter.

I walked out without getting fries. Or a veggie burger. Or a Coke. I don't know if I will ever go back.

It was a good feeling. I sat in my car, breathing deeply for a moment, staring at the door I had just closed, and then I see a child, a boy of maybe 10 or 11, waddle to it. He must have been at least twice the size he should be for his weight. "I'll bet his mother is fat too," I thought, both sad and angry for him, bursting out of his much-too-small sweatpants, rolls of fat pouring out of his clothes. He looked happy going into Burger King, but I'll bet he wasn't happy overall. I know how fat kids are treated. I was one, and I wasn't even anywhere near his size. Maybe that's why he's not in school today. Maybe they pulled him out of school because of bullying. Fat shaming.

His "fat mother" came next, only it was actually a fat father, the same shape as his child, too-right jeans squeezing his belly over and down them. Our eyes met. I smiled, so he wouldn't know what I was really thinking. One of the things I was thinking was "shame on me for automatically blaming the mother."

I drove home to heat up an Amy's vegan burrito and make a smoothie rich with fruits, veggies, and seeds. Proud.

Thought of my eleventh-grade year, when I worked at Burger

King. Food was deducted from our meager paychecks, but that didn't stop me from cramming a fish sandwich, large fries, and especially a large chocolate milkshake (extra chocolate, since I made them) down my throat every day. Thank God I escaped that place. In eleventh grade. And today.

September 18, Friday

Weight: 156.1
Ate: : Smoothie, Amy's burrito, ½ cup dark chocolate covered almonds, 6 peanut butter crackers, dinner of rice, veggies, soy sauce, and sweet potato fries
Exercise: Dog walk: 14,528 steps

Rethinking Fat Shaming "Humor"

I still don't agree with YouTube censoring a fat shaming video, but on the other hand, I took a look at the Nicole Arbour video again and thought, "Why should we be so mean to each other?"

Personally, and may she rest in peace, I never liked Joan Rivers' humor. I guess it was consider "okay" in the 1970s and '80s, when I watched her on Johnny Carson, to use women's body sizes (especially poor Elizabeth Taylor) as the source of jokes. She wasn't the only one of course.

But I, the teenager and then young woman watching her and listening to her berate women for their body size, flinched. It was mean. It seemed wrong to make a living off someone else's "failure," which perhaps we can look at Liz's weight gain as, although I don't think that's right either. (You can search for Joan's Elizabeth Taylor jokes online; they are too cruel to even include here.)

In any case, I only watched her because I loved Johnny Carson. His was the humor I liked: warm, self-deprecating, never attacking others. Isn't that the richest kind of comedy of all? I don't recall him using women's bodies as the source of his jokes although it didn't go unnoticed to me that his various string of wives were all *thin*. Of course. Something else I could cross of my list of possibilities in life: dating a celebrity. I already knew, at 12 years old, maybe 5 to 10 pounds overweight, that I was too fat for that lifestyle. I was *not good enough*. That attitude has carried throughout my life, so that when I dated men, most of them were the wrong kind of men, losers, cruel, unemployed, whatever…but they wanted to date me. A fat chick. So I was grateful. What a waste of time. And life.

September 19, Saturday

Weight: No weigh in; at the writers' conference
Ate: : Oatmeal with peanut butter, hummus sandwich, ½ cup dark chocolate covered almonds peanut butter crackers, ¼ cup almonds
Exercise: 10,721 steps

Social Square Revisited

A few friends messaged or emailed me asking if I was okay. So maybe I'm actually missed on the social square, or my absence has been noticed. I'm sure I will eventually return to posting and reading posts, responding to people. It was a source of human interaction of sorts that I had every day.

But I guess I'm a state of being alone in my grief, and in my healing, from losing my dog, Chewie. Instead of the word "dog" I was trying to think of what word explains how close we were, but no words and all words worked; a dog can encompass so many roles in our lives: best friend, child, parent, guide, gift, but most of all, just love, in its purest simplest form. Love. I miss her love.

September 20, Sunday

Weight: Just walking around hotel
Ate: Oatmeal with peanut butter, hummus sandwich, peanut butter crackers, ¼ cup almonds, ¼ cup seeds, smoothie, Amy's dinner, 1 giant bag of popcorn (no butter)
Exercise: Just walking around hotel: 12,116 steps

Anorexia

Although I have had periods of starving myself in my life, when I was younger (and dumber?), I can't see myself ever being anorexic.

For one thing, I like food too much. And I dislike hunger.

Fortunately, I think one reason this diet is working, slowly but surely, is that I am not eating foods I blazingly *love*. I had no control over foods I loved, meaning cakes, cookies, ice cream, and candy bars. Now I know what it is like to eat slowly, to live simply, to let go of addictions and obsessions. Even food ones. Especially food ones.

September 21, Monday

Weight: 156.9
Ate: Smoothie, 1 Amy's frozen burrito
Exercise: Dog walks: 14,425 steps

Epic Fail?

Last night was a shocker, because, clothed and after drinking a smoothie, the scale said 160. This is why you don't weigh yourself at night. I vowed never to see the 160s again, but there it was. I vow to work harder!

I spent the Friday through Sunday at a hotel in Anchorage at a conference. Here's one thing I learned being away: the daily dog walks and writing down food are important. The daily (morning!) weigh-in is essential.

Why? Because I didn't get any "tough" exercise, and I ate too much.

In my "old" days, I always lost weight when I travelled. I think it's because I have less stress when I'm away from home (which is also my office). This time away was important, because I needed to "break" from home and the loss of Chewie for a few days. I return a little stronger, a little better, but also a little fatter. I'll take care of that. Quickly! So I'm off to dog walk #2 for the day.

Later: Did the second walk. Good for me. But the reason I call today's topic "Epic Fail" is because I actually weigh more than I did at the beginning of this month, 3 weeks ago! That is not good! I already know what I need to do…I'm just dreading doing it. Go to the gym. Start weight lifting. Doing more muscle work. Yuck. But a "necessary evil" that I will come to love, right? At least to like. Sigh.

September 22, Tuesday

Weight: 155.9
Ate: 2 smoothies, Amy's frozen breakfast meal, bowl of oatmeal with chocolate and peanut butter, ¼ cup of almonds
Exercise: Dog walk: 11,531 steps

TOPS Gain

For only the third time this year, I gained weight from the previous week's weigh-in at TOPS. This week's weigh-in showed an astounding 2.2 pounds gained. Not good. Need to get a hold of this. But after a dog walk, I spent most of the day in bed. I think I am very depressed, from Chewie's death, from gaining weight, from fall (and the threat of winter), from Kip's behavioral issues, from my son's increasing anger at me (he's 15, and I'm a mom; it's not like it wasn't expected?), and from the increase in fibromyalgia pain lately.

But there's another reason: the writers' conference. What a depressing 3 days of negativity that was. Last year I came out inspired and willing to "quit my day job" and go for the dream, but now I wonder if anyone still reads and if agents could be any crueler. One said he gets 13,000 queries a year but only accepts 7. What?

I am finally living my dream, and maybe I wasn't really worried whether I'd make it or not; just the fact that one or two books sell a day seemed like an incredible victory for me over a year ago, when I had none available. But then the stock market has been crashing; the hard work I've done earning and saving all that is starting to look like it's wasted (again), and I question whether I will be able to stay out of the job market long enough to write a best seller.

So tragedy, depression, pain, and fear…no wonder I gained 2.2 pounds and stayed in bed all day.

September 23, Wednesday

Weight: 156.5
Ate: veggie quesadillas, hash browns, Diet Coke, hummus with carrots, Amy's burrito, smoothie, ¼ cup almonds, ¼ cup sunflower seeds, 1 large vegan cookie
Exercise: Dog walk: 11,531 steps

Company

Wonderful day spent with my niece; one day left of her visit. I will miss her. I will not miss the food. For some reason, it's easier for me to diet when I am alone and friendless.

September 24, Thursday

Weight: 157.8
Ate: Smoothie, small popcorn, Taco Bell 5-layer burrito, 2 bowls vegan spaghetti with veggies, ¼ cup dried strawberries
Exercise: Dog walk: 11,280 steps

Uh-oh, Spaghettio

How the weight piles on so fast and furious. Now I'm up 5 pounds from my lowest point this year, this month. I'm frightened, but I'm also aware that I can get back to my boring routine now that my niece has left, although I will miss her terribly. I will also be able to be hungry and starve as necessary to get these 5 pounds off without the temptation of going out to eat (or asking her bring me home a giant tub of popcorn when she went to the movies…me bad!).

Here's what I know about a weight-gain "slump." In my case, it's usually related to one of more of the following:

- Depression (losing Chewie)
- Stress (too much work usually, but not so in this case; however, the stock market plunge and my son's issues of late have been stressful, plus worries about Kip's behavior and winter's coming)
- Surgeries, injuries, or pain (in this case, the fibromyalgia flare-up of the last few weeks has been intense)

Here's what else I know:

- I have come too far and worked to hard to lose this weight to give up.
- I will reach my goal. Even if I have to reconfigure what that goal is for now. Maybe my body will just settle in the mid- to low-150s for a time, and that's still an incredible victory from last year's high of 240!
- I will continue to be vegan.
- I will continue to walk the dogs most if not every day (weekends I'm hesitant now because of the number of people on the trails).

So I decide to be not upset by the number on the scale but instead challenged, motivated, and encouraged that this is just my typical bounce before a fall. A warning to decrease the food a bit, burn a few more calories. I'll get there. I'll be okay.

September 25, Friday

Weight: 157.5
Ate: 2 smoothies, ¼ cup almonds, Amy's meal, 1 giant popcorn (no butter) at movie theater, humus with carrots
Exercise: Dog walk (forgot Fitbit: 5,000 steps), plus gym: 10,000 total (estimated)

Walking vs. Gyms

Just finished a walk on the trails with the dogs. Was surprised that I wasn't worried about bears munching on me after watching feeding time with the blacks and grizzlies at Alaska Wildlife Conservation Center last night. While watching them chew frozen pig ribs like I used to eat M&Ms, I envisioned my family and friends giggling at my funeral because of the irony of an animal rights activist being taken down by the animals she loved. And I imagined how my dogs chased the bear right to me before my demise. Sigh. Old Yeller, they're not! Miza was, but now he's getting too old and crippled. I pictured him jogging for home while the bear was crunching my arm, looking back as if to say: "I'll let them know you're in trouble!"

Anyway, I am really just telling you all this to delay going to the gym.

Later: Back from the gym. I believe it would take a major change in my personality to "enjoy" going to the gym. Pretty much, I was an epic fail. I'm so bored and slightly disgusted and very uncomfortable in gyms. So there we go. Not a match for my personality. While Greg spent the hour running on the treadmill, I attempted to work out with the weight machines, having to put the weights on the lowest settings because of the fibromyalgia pain.

The best part of the gym, as far as I was concerned, was leaving it. So I'm home now, running a bath, happy.

September 26, Saturday

Weight: 158
Ate: Smoothie; about 5 cups of spaghetti with olives, olive oil, tomatoes, garlic, and pesto mix; dark chocolate covered almonds (about ½ cup)
Exercise: Dog walk: 13,164 steps

Weight Gain

Wow, really up. 7 pounds up from my lowest point this month. I know a couple pounds of this is the salty popcorn I ate late last night at the movies.

Also, I haven't told you this, but I have been taking pain pills again, which cause constipation. I had my 6-month appointment with my thyroid doctor and admitted how much I am suffering from the fibromyalgia pain. She prescribed pain meds. Yesterday is the first time ever (except maybe right after surgery) that I took two in one day. The pain is maddening. I woke up in agony today, but of course I haven't taken any as I want to drive today. Not sure how long I can hold out. It's miserable.

The pain pills help with the pain, but they cause me to be "plugged up," so that's not good. Speaking of that, I have included my thoughts after watching a documentary about Elvis.

Elvis and Healthy Digestion

Watched a scary documentary about Elvis's death at 42: *Autopsy: The Last Hours of: Elvis Presley.* We've all heard heart attack, obesity, cardiac arrhythmia, drugs. But the most surprising information in it to me was about his bowels. Perhaps TMI (respect the dead, for gosh sakes), but it is still important to consider for our own health. I guess, since I've always had "problems" in this area, even as a baby (and so did my son), I'm especially interested in it.

According to Medical Bag ("Features"), Dr. George Nichopoulos said in *The King and Dr. Nick*, "chronic constipation killed Elvis":

> *In a 2010* Fox News *interview, he stated, "We didn't realize until the autopsy that his constipation was as bad-we knew it was because it was hard for us to treat, but we didn't realize what it had done."*
>
> *According his autopsy, the diameter of Elvis's colon was 5 to 6 inches, which is about double the size of the typical person's, and instead of being 4 to 5 feet long, his colon was 8 to 9 feet in length.*
>
> *"We found stool in his colon which had been there for four or five months because of the poor motility of the bowel."*
>
> *Nichopoulos noted that Elvis had inherited a condition called bowel paralysis, which made defecating difficult.*

The documentary described the stool as grey, clay-like matter. I can't seem to get that image out of my mind. How awful. How agonizing to try to "go." It made me think of his diet, probably rich in everything but vegetables...lots of meat and sugar. I remember how much trouble I had as a child, especially, before going vegetarian. I would go weeks without being able to "go." When I did go, it was agony. I thought my insides were being ripped out. "Elvis, Elvis, I get you!" I want to tell him. "I understand!" And it's the kind of thing you can't talk about with anyone, even your doctor.

In fact, my dad might have saved my life. He knew about my issue because one time I ended up in an emergency room in Seattle when we were all there. Everyone thought I had appendicitis because I was in so much pain, but no, ma'am, you're just plugged up from top to bottom. I feel like I've been "plugged up" most of my life.

My poor dad died of colon cancer, but before he died, he told me his doctor recommended Senokot, which advertises itself as a natural vegetable laxative. I have no problem with taking one a day as needed, several times a week. I wish Elvis had had some.

For more on healthy vs. unhealthy stools, search online, or see the link to Robynne Chutkan's article on DoctorOz.com (in Works Cited list).

Goal Weight

In the past 15 years, since my child was born, I have been to the mid- to high 150s, aiming for the mid- or low 140s, three times, and I have failed to get to the 140s. Maybe, at 55 years old, forced menopause, with thyroid issues, the 150s is all I should plan for. Maybe I should make 153 (my healthywage.com goal) my actual "goal," for TOPS, for me, and be satisfied. (And then, if I happen to go into the 140s because of my lifestyle changes, yay!)

This thought has been in my mind throughout the entire journey.

What happens when I get to the 150s? What will be different this time?

I thought I could add more weights, but the fibromyalgia pain is making that seem impossible, at least for now, through this long drawn-out painful Alaskan fall. If I hopped a plane to Hawaii and beach walked the next 2 or 3 weeks, I have a feeling I'd come back at least 10 pounds lighter. But I have a child (who currently hates me), dogs, Greg, little income....I don't want to go to Hawaii. Alone. To lose weight.

So here I am, at a standstill. Clearly, I need to do something different than I have been doing the last few weeks. Yes I'm in mourning (for Chewie), yes I'm stressed (my son and my pup Kip), yes my dream has been blown (from the writers' conference), yes I hurt (fibromyalgia hell), yes I'm hungry (fattening up for winter like an old grizzly?), yes I'm lazy (I want to stay in bed where it's warm and soft and safe), yes I am out of nicotine gum (sigh, but still over 19 weeks cigarette-free), yes...I have excuses galore.

But I am also fiercely determined not to gain this weight back.

I'm going to "settle" on 153. That gives me a reasonable, reachable goal. Achievable by the TOPS Fall Rally on October 3. Here's hoping it's enough to win me the "State Queen" title and a trip to Orlando next year. In any case, I am healthier, fitter, stronger than a year ago.

September 27, Sunday

Weight: 159
Ate: Smoothie, avocado, ¼ cup sunflower seeds,. 4 slices of Tofurky with vegetable chips
Exercise: Dog walk: 5,766 steps

No Way – Not Giving Up!

Even though I wrote yesterday that I'm going to "settle" on 153, and even though I gained another pound from yesterday (up almost 7 in the last 2 weeks), the thought of giving up depressed me and infuriated me.

No, I'm not giving up! I will not give in. I will reach my goal.

I will figure this out.

September 28, Monday

Weight: 156.3
Ate: Smoothie, hummus with about 20 vegetable chips, 4 slices of
Tofurky with vegetable chips
Exercise: None: 2,062 steps

My Body Is a Cage

I heard this Arcade Fire song on the show *House* (actually it was a Peter Gabrielle version):

> *My body is a cage that keeps me*
>
> *From dancing with the one I love*
>
> *But my mind holds the key*

It is haunting, beautiful, and sang by someone who sounds in both mental and physical anguish.

Which is how I feel today.

The pain was so intense, I barely got out of bed at all. I certainly didn't make a dog walk. The dogs seemed understanding, as dogs are, even the rascally puppies. I didn't take a pain pill. I suffered. Watched bad TV. Moaned. And didn't eat much. I hurt too much to eat.

> *Set my spirit free*
>
> *Set my spirit free*

– Arcade Fire, "My Body Is A Cage"

September 29, Tuesday

Weight: 156.1
Ate: 2 smoothies, 3 peanuts (in shells), 1 Amy's frozen meal, oatmeal
with peanut butter and chocolate protein powder
Exercise: Dog walk: 10,740 steps

Lucky Break

If I'm lucky and vigilant, I will lose another pound by tomorrow, which will make this a "break even" month. Not a good thing, when you're trying to lose weight.

What ups and downs this month has been! How happy I was to see 152 on the scale, and then how mortified to see it climb right back up to 159. How my confidence has been demolished. Yet still, I seek the goal...about 145. I still believe I'll get there. Somehow.

And I miss Chewie.

September 30, Wednesday

Weight: 157.1
Ate: Large bowl of lentil and veggies soup, 1 vegan cookie, 2 smoothies, 2 slices of Tofurky.
Exercise: Dog walk: 10,000 steps
Inches: Chest: 42.5 Waist: 37.50 Hips: 40.5
Body Fat %: 43.12 BMI: 27

What I Did Right and Wrong This Month

Overall, I experimented this month with eating "normally," meaning, I tried not being an a "diet" to see what happened. What happened was that I didn't lose and in fact gained weight. So even when I do shift to "normal" eating after reaching goal, it will need to be less than what I consumed this month. Or I will need to do more exercise.

What I have done right is:

- Stayed vegan
- Exercised almost every day (dog walks) except during the conference
- Went to the gym (but only once!)
- Did not turn to eating too much after the loss of my beloved dog Chewie. (But I lost my energy.)
- Forgave myself for not doing as well as I wanted to; accepted that I am in mourning.
- Saw I had a huge gain (7 pounds!) from my lowest number this month, so for the last few days, I cut back on eating a bit.

What I have done wrong is:

- I didn't lose weight, for the first time. Worse, I gained 2 pounds! I started the month at 155.1 pounds and ended it at 157.1 pounds. During the month, I dropped to 152, but then went up to 159.
- I slowed down quite a bit on the walks due to fibromyalgia pain and depression (losing Chewie).
- I didn't walk at all or move at all one day due to pain.
- I only went to the gym once. I didn't do weightlifting because of the fibromyalgia, as well as because I'm just that plain lazy.
- I ate too much. Ultimately, that's what it comes down to, right? I ate too much considering the exercise I did. I took too many calories in. Epic fail.

OCTOBER

Weight: 157.1
Exercise: 10,000 steps a day average, PLUS weight lifting at least 3 times per week
Inches: Chest: 41.5 Waist: 35 Hips: 40.5
Body Fat %: 42.75 BMI: 27
Motivation: To reach HealthyWage.com goal and win the $ this month (October 10 – 24 is "weigh out" time) and receive KOPS status at TOPS (I'm thinking about 152 I'll call it good, as I can still lose 7 pounds from there and be in "KOPS" status, so down to 145, if I were that lucky.) This is MY MONTH! To ACHIEVE! EVERYTHING!

October 1, Thursday

Weight: 157.1
Ate: 3 smoothies, 5 chips, 2 slices Tofurky, Diet Coke, ½ cup sunflower seeds, 1 avocado, 2 bananas, ¼ cup peanut butter, 5 carrots
Exercise: Dog walk: 12,568 steps

A New Beginning

Well, the good news is my waist went down 2.5 inches since yesterday. That was some swollen belly! So as far as inches go in September, I basically stayed the same, except for losing 1 inch off my breasts (of course, so unfair).

Feeling good today; feeling strong; the pain has subsided, even though the temperatures are below freezing, which is why my beginning of the month picture looks like this at left: Okay, on the right is one without the hat and coat (and with the addition of the Pup Who Loves Me: Kip).

October is a new beginning for me. I know what I have to do: eat less, exercise more. Do better. Be better. Lift some weights.

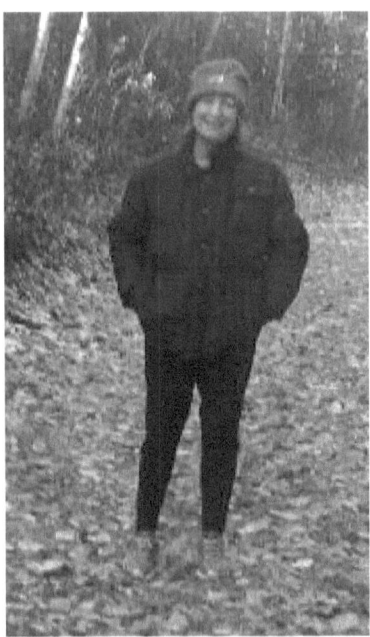 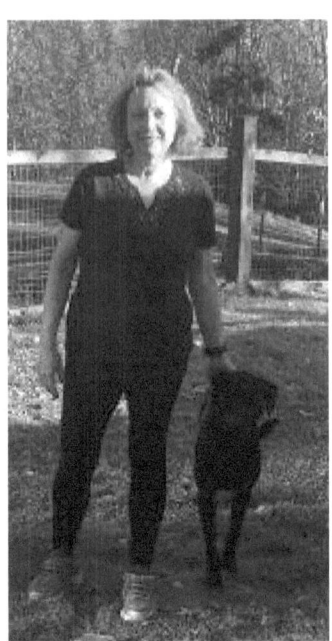

Photos of me today.

October 2, Friday

Weight: 157.7
Ate: Amy's burrito, 2 smoothies, ½ cup dark chocolate covered almonds,
1 cup of soup
Exercise: Dog walk: 11,680 steps

Umpqua Community College (UCC)

Another school shooting yesterday. All of them are tragic and terrible and ridiculously wrong, but this one was personal. For 4 or 5 years of my graduate school life, I drove the 45 miles from my cabin to teach at a beautiful little community college near the grand Umpqua River. Everyone was nice to me there. I slaved away for the tiny paycheck of a part-time English teacher and tried to get hired full time. By the time an opening came up, I was exhausted, tired, getting burned out from teaching at three colleges, working editing jobs, and going to grad school (not to mention being in a relationship from hell). It was between two of us, and sweet Diane got the job. I didn't know if she was a better teacher than I was, but I knew she deserved it for another reason. She "looked" the part: tall, slim, smiling, stylish. While I, a poor graduate student who had still managed to find the funds to stuff 50 pounds on my body that last dissertation year, dressed frumpy and fat (so how could I possibly get such a Great Job?), was running scared, was needing to escape Oregon and an abusive relationship. I loved all my co-workers, but they made the right choice. I was meant to get out of dodge, so to speak, and so I did.

But yesterday, I mourned that beautiful campus and community. I called the friends I still had, over 22 years later, former students I am still close to. I thought of the happy, sunny days there. I thought of the rain that scared me so much while driving home, when the "triples" (three long trailers attached to a semi truck) went by, leaving me driving blind. I thought of the deep dark fog that sometimes obscured my drive…but still I only missed one class. All for about $1 an hour, based on how much time grading and prep and commuting took me.

The reason I missed one class was because of my Ph.D. Field Exams, which took 2 days. I had explained to my students why there wouldn't be class on Friday; that I would be spending 4 hours a day taking essay exams to see if I qualified for the Ph.D. program. When I walked into the before-exam UCC class, the entire table at the front of the room was covered in bags of M&Ms. My sweet UCC students had bought me my favorite food to munch on during the exam. So sweet!

I thought of how just three summers ago I drove my son to UCC, driving him to the campus, but I was too embarrassed to get out of the car to go see my former colleagues because I was so fat. So we didn't go into Snyder Hall, where my department was, my office was, and many of my classrooms were. Where I spent hours of my life. Where sometimes, when the abuser was especially bad, I'd drive to in the middle of the night and sleep on the couch, my dogs with me, sneaking them out early before anyone else arrived.

It was the only place I felt safe.

Yesterday was not a safe place at Umpqua, or that same Snyder Hall. Yesterday I mourned for a campus now forever bloodied and changed by a stupid mad man. Yesterday, I cried for a UCC I knew and that will never be again.

(And related to this book, yesterday, I ate way too much.)

October 3, Saturday

Weight: 157.3
Ate: 2 smoothies, ½ cup dark chocolate covered almonds, 1 cup of soup, 1 large unbuttered popcorn, 1 Diet Pepsi, 1 baked potato with fresh veggies
Exercise: Dog walk: 11,546 steps

Popcorn

I'm at the movies, slamming popcorn and Diet Pepsi down my throat, wondering what the heck I am doing and why can't I watch a movie at a movie theater without munching my way through it? It's purely habit. I've changed other habits. I'm going to have to change this one. Next time, no matter what the sign says about no outside food or drinks, I'm bringing baggies of veggies, some hummus, and a water bottle. Done.

October 4, Sunday

Weight: 157.7
Ate: 3 smoothies, 1 Amy's burrito, 1 cup of soup
Exercise: Dog walk: 10,397 steps

Grief

I am overwhelmed with sadness since the UCC murders. I don't get it. I try to bond with my son, but he's having none of it. He is upset over the New Rules in the House until he gets his grades up. His addiction to Minecraft is destroying his chances for college or a future. But as a parent who loves him, I am always so torn at this act of taking away his computer, which is also most of his social life. I feel like a Giant Parent Fail. I have so little energy to do what I should, to be different than I am. Why can't he be happy reading books, writing stories, walking his dog...like I was? What is this crazed computerized world about? In our glee to connect, are we really all disconnecting? Forever?

October 5, Monday

Weight: 157
Ate: 2 smoothies, 2 Amy's burritos, ¼ cup pumpkin sees, 1 bowl of oatmeal with peanut butter and chocolate
Exercise: Dog walk: 12,248 steps

Depression

There are so many reasons I have fallen into the smog of depression right now:

- The UCC shooting – it's personal, because I worked there, loved it, and felt safe there.
- My son is treating me poorly; he is furious that I limited his computer to 2 hours a day 3 days a week until the grades are up.
- Greg is treating me poorly. Meaning, he's crabby. I make him crabby. Whatever.
- I am grieving Chewie's loss.
- I am worried about my son beyond belief – his health, his grades, his future.
- I can't seem to focus on work, even though I finally have some reports to do.
- I am not making any money, well – 35 cents a day from book sales – yikes!
- The stock market has been plummeting the last 2 weeks, so I am afraid about all I've saved and invested to allow me to take this time off from work to write.
- Ever since the writers' conference, I have lost my faith and excitement about writing; the future of books seems bleak, and it's hard to even consider all the work involved in

writing a book to see it sit there unsold.

- I guess I'm probably lonely; I don't have many friends, especially here in Alaska.
- I have 5 days to reach 153.7 pounds (with clothes on) for HealthyWage.com. Of course, the weigh-in runs till October 24, so I'm not really worried about achieving this, but still…. It looms.

Later: I drove to a counseling center, was turned away, drove to another one, stopped on the way at Walmart for dog food, roamed the aisles to get Fitbit steps and pick up items, bought muffins for my son (so I could see the hint of a smile when he got home, which I did), felt a little better after strolling around the store, then went to the other counseling center. Tried to explain my depression to the emergency walk-in guy; he determined I was "only" a level 1, so I was shuffled to the appointment counter some 2 weeks away. Still, it felt better to talk to an actual person, if only briefly, about UCC and having a teenager and losing Chewie. Even if, I felt, he didn't understand how important Chewie was to me. At least I took steps toward healing, even if I have to wait 2 weeks to see someone.

One thing I thought of during the 30-minute drive to the second counseling center is that in the "old days" before the "New Me" I would have dulled my throbbing depression and anxiety with a cigarette. And some M&Ms and Hershey's Kisses. That's how I staved off the beast of depression before, and it worked. I felt a little sorry for the old me, really only fat and a smoker because I was self-medicating.

Now I have to find other, healthier ways of coping. With life. And death.

October 6, Tuesday

Weight: 155.2
Ate: 2 smoothies, 2 coffees, 1 soup, chocolate "pudding" (peanut butter, 1 avocado, chocolate protein powder, cocoa powder, ice, and water)

Exercise: Two dog walks: 18,105 steps

Not Like Normal People

Nice drop of 2 pounds since yesterday. The only thing I really did differently was some weight lifting. So that makes sense. I already know I need more exercise in my life; I'm just dreading it. But I manage to "Fitbit" my way to 10,000 steps most days, sometimes by pacing the last 1,500 in front of my TV. The last couple nights I added weights to my stroll, pumping 5-pound beasts in various ways.

"I'm not like 'normal' people," I remind myself, from books gone by. "I need to exercise more and eat less than most." That is just the way my life is. So I accept it and go on.

October 7, Wednesday

Weight: 155.5
Ate: Amy's burrito, 2 smoothies, carrots, avocado, 1 can of soup
Exercise: Dog walk: 16,063 steps

Short-Burst Diet

Dr. Oz, on yesterday's show, discussed the 5-days a month, 1,000-calories a day "fast" that I discussed previously, after a study suggested it would have health benefits. He calls it the "short-burst diet." There is a link on his site to the video, but not (yet?) to the recipes (which were all plant-based; I'm especially eager to see the tofu chocolate mousse!). However, I challenged a TOPS member to try it with me for the next 5 days. Basically, I'll just try to keep my calories to 1,000 or under for 5 days, and see what happens. I've got the HealthyWage.com weigh-in Saturday!

October 8, Thursday

Weight: 156.5
Ate: 4 small bags (150 calories each) of chocolate-covered almonds, 1 veggie burger, 1 smoothie, 1 vegetarian hot dog (no bun)
Exercise: Dog walk: 20,412 steps

50% Trick

Dr. Oz had an interesting suggestion on Tuesday's show. He said your waist should be half your height. He suggested it's preferable to BMI. That means at 64 inches, I should have a 32-inch waist. I'm 3 inches from that, and that actually makes sense. That's how much I'd like to lose.

However, during yesterday's show, Dr. Oz used a string, cut it in two, people stood on it (which probably added several inches); therefore, he "made it fit" for someone in the audience who looked like she carried too much around the middle. I'm going with the 50% of your height instead of the string trick. It's more accurate.

October 9, Friday

Weight: 156.6
Ate: 2 small bags (150 calories each) of chocolate-covered almonds, 1 bag of cashews (160 calories), 1 slice of Good Seed bread with hummus, 2 smoothies, 1 Amy's burrito, 1 vegetarian hot dog (no bun)
Exercise: Dog walk: 12,668 steps

Thyroid Grrr

Okay, so my weight is going the wrong way for tomorrow's HealthyWage.com weigh-out. Crapola! Fortunately, I have from October 10 to the 24 to meet the 153.6 goal. It was always in my mind to step on the scale the first day of the weigh-out, though, with Total Victory.

Anyway, that's not going to happen. But I have been working out hard (really upped the steps this week, plus weight lifting!) and dieting pretty strictly, so I'm not blaming myself for anything. I'm doing the right things. Okay, maybe the dark chocolate-covered almonds yesterday weren't necessary, but they were a comfort food after I found out I have to have another surgery. In my neck. My lovely little thyroid tumor, that has been floating around in there and been checked and ultrasounded and biopsied for the last 14 years, is getting larger and uglier, so it gets to come out. And I get an overnight in the hospital.

The doc tried to schedule it for Monday, but I looked on my calendar and my glasses come in Monday. Since the puppies ate another pair, I've been going blindly through the world, only able to read with difficulty, so I said, "Make it the next Monday, the 19th. I'll have my glasses by then and can read while I'm in the hospital for hours waiting for my surgery to begin and after."

Reading has taken over TV viewing and Internet time-wasting in my life, thankfully. That's the good news.

Another good news item is the surgery: I guess I've never wanted this tumor, nor to take Synthroid, and I certainly never want to go through a painful biopsy again, so I'm happy to see it go. (But I'm a little bit scared, too, I'll admit only to you.)

October 10, Saturday

Weight: 155.2
Ate: 1 coffee with chocolate "greens," smoothie, and all kinds of vegan foods at Organic Oasis restaurant in Anchorage: chocolate cake, 2 cookies, hummus with pita bread, garlic, and olive oil; and a pasta with pesto and lime dinner
Exercise: Dog walk: 10.902 steps

HealthyWage Weigh-in Day

Oh golly gee. 1.6 pounds over. On my scale. Under on my son's scale (but it's different every time), and only 1 pound over on Greg's scale, which seems to match the TOPS scale for weights. So close! I could starve and not drink today, but instead, I'm just going to keep trying, eat a little less, move a little more.

I had no energy yesterday; after the dog walk, I couldn't even do work, type my diary, or exercise. I stayed in bed all day. I don't think starving is the right concept. I feel like I hardly eat anything, and yet I'm still well over my 1,200-calorie-a-day goal (and 1,000-day-goal for the 5-day burst diet). How do people live like this?

We were on the trails today, and I asked for a compliment from Greg. He said, "You look enticing."

"Enticing." I rolled the word over my tongue. It's a great

word. But all I could think of while saying it was chocolate cake.

October 11, Sunday

Weight: 157.7
Ate: 2 smoothies, 3 small bowls of angel-hair pasta with tons of veggies and pesto and olive oil, 1 vegan burger with veggies, ½ Diet Coke, ¼ cup sunflower seeds
Exercise: Dog walk: 10,410 steps

Oasis?

So, Saturday and Sunday I had amazing vegan foods at a restaurant in Anchorage called Organic Oasis. In fact, Saturday, I was so overwhelmed by the choices (which I usually never have at restaurants in the Valley), I chose four items: cookies, cake, pasta with pesto, and hummus with pita bread.

Not a great idea since I'm trying to reach my HealthyWage goal this week of 153.6, and now I'm up to 157.7. What is wrong with me?

Well, I hardly ever go to Anchorage, so it was in the spirit of having such an amazing selection of healthy, vegan foods. Then my wonderful brother, the doctor, made me my favorite pesto pasta filled with fresh veggies. Which I ate and ate and ate. Finally, I took the giant bowl and separated it into plates and froze it, moving it all down to Greg's freezer. Out of sight; out of mind. It does work.

Anyway, I'm wondering if this eating "frenzy" (which is really probably just normal eating for normal people) is my fear about the upcoming thyroid surgery. I know I'm scared, but I'm ignoring it by distracting myself with TV, food, whatever.

October 12, Monday

Weight: 158.1
Ate: Coffee, water, 1 small smoothie, 1 cup of soup, and 2 cups of vegetable broth
Exercise: Dog walk: 13,587 steps

Up Again

I guess I am going to have to do something drastic this week, like try the Master Cleanse or some other torture. I don't want to do this the week before the scary surgery, where he's going to basically cut my throat to rip out half my thyroid. I don't want to starve.

On the other hand, I don't want to come this far and lose my HealthyWage money. Crap.

October 13, Tuesday

Weight: 156.1
Ate: 1 bag of cashews (150 calories), 1 smoothie, 1 bowl of pea soup, 1 small plate of pesto pasta with veggies
Exercise: Dog walk: 14,439 steps

And Down Again

You know, the concept of the 500- or 1,000-calorie a day "fast" for a few days is great. I already know it is about all that ultimately works for me to drop a few pounds. Is my weight loss all really about a few days of semi-starvation followed by a few weeks of "normal" eating? Perhaps.

In any case, yesterday I had one small smoothie, 1 cup of soup, and 2 cups of vegetable broth. That's all. Still came to about 850 calories. Let's face it: I eat too much most of the time. And I'm not the only one.

October 14, Wednesday

Weight: 155.9
Ate: 2 smoothies, 1 small plate of pesto pasta, about 5 peanuts, 1 small bag of cashews
Exercise: Dog walk: 15,402 steps

Trying Harder

Walking hard, eating less, to try to meet the HealthyWage.com goal before I go into surgery Monday, just in case something happens to me...I want my family to have the money. (Not that I'm nervous about having my throat cut and my thyroid ripped out or anything!)

It's not fun to have to "diet" the week before, in the back of your mind, you think, this might be my last. I've also taken on some tedious formatting work. I think it's the caretaker side of me…wanting to make sure my family is comfortable.

I'm thinking maybe 2 more days of semi-starvation (that's what I call under 1,000 calories a day; Dr. Oz calls it the "short burst diet," and the University of Southern California calls it the Fasting Mimicking Diet (FMD). Fortunately, 5 days a month of cutting calories drastically is supposed to help you in many ways: "reduced biomarkers" linked to aging, diabetes, cancer and heart disease. Oh yes, and less body fat.

When I try to restrict down to 1,000 calories a day I realize that I eat way more calories normally than I think I do (and I'm sure I'm not alone on this). I "try" to keep them around 1,500, but I rarely count, and generally have no idea. The Fitbit app is helpful, as I scan UPC codes right into the phone and it tells me how many calories I'm consuming (but you've got to watch those servings; one cup of instant soup is one serving to me, but two servings on its container, so you have to add two of them if you drink one…very frustrating and confusing).

Usually by the time I've had my smoothie of banana (102 calories), avocado (234), pumpkin seeds (95), chia seeds (138), protein powder (130), various frozen fruits (65-150), kale or spinach (14-50), and carrots (50 for two), I've already consumed at least 650 calories! (When I say "two smoothies," I mean that huge blended drink…it fills up two 32-ounce cups.) And that's usually by 9 a.m. So I've got 12 hungry hours to go.

October 15, Thursday

Weight: 152.8
Ate: 1 smoothie, 1 small plate of pesto pasta, small order sweet potato fries, tortilla with fresh veggies, oatmeal with chocolate and peanut

butter, 2 more plates of pesto pasta (finished my brother's gift, finally!)
Exercise: Dog walk: 9,757 (on iPhone pedometer; forgot Fitbit); plus
3,748 steps on Fitbit
Inches: Chest: 40.5 Waist: 35.25 Hips: 41
Body Fat %: 27.34 BMI: 26-2/9

Victory!

Made it to HealthyWage.com weight! Won the $! Uploading the video now.

Gosh, I work well under a deadline! I really came through in the last few days, taking 10,000-step hard dog walks through the woods (instead of 5,000-step ones) and keeping my calories just under 1,000 a day.

Hungry, grumpy, and down 6 pounds since Monday (gotta say the short-burst diet – at least my version of it since there were no recipes online – works!). I'll take it!

Later: Read about the planned destruction of more of my favorite trails by the borough. Made me so depressed, mostly because I love and value those trails that the borough is turning into a garbage dump. And for another thing because I can't imagine how I'm going to get the "bad puppies" to the maze of unused tiny trails I discovered without going that way...the blocked trail that no one uses. I fear my ability to get in a good hour or so of exercise every day will tank because of it. And without exercise...you and I both know what will happen to me.

I took myself to bed most of the afternoon. Researched solutions. Told the borough what I thought of their evil plan (useless; I've told them for 14 years). Then found a puppy group; was honest about the mental state of my pups, begged them to let me try Harper only this weekend; most said okay. If I can just get my puppies to learn to behave around strange dogs...please God.

In any case, I won today! I wanted to get that done before the surgery, so in case something goes wrong, my family will get the prize money: Here's what HealthyWage emailed: *"You are set and a winner. Congratulations on your weight loss."* (Okay, they misspelled "congratulations," but I corrected that. I worked hard for this; I want it perfect!)

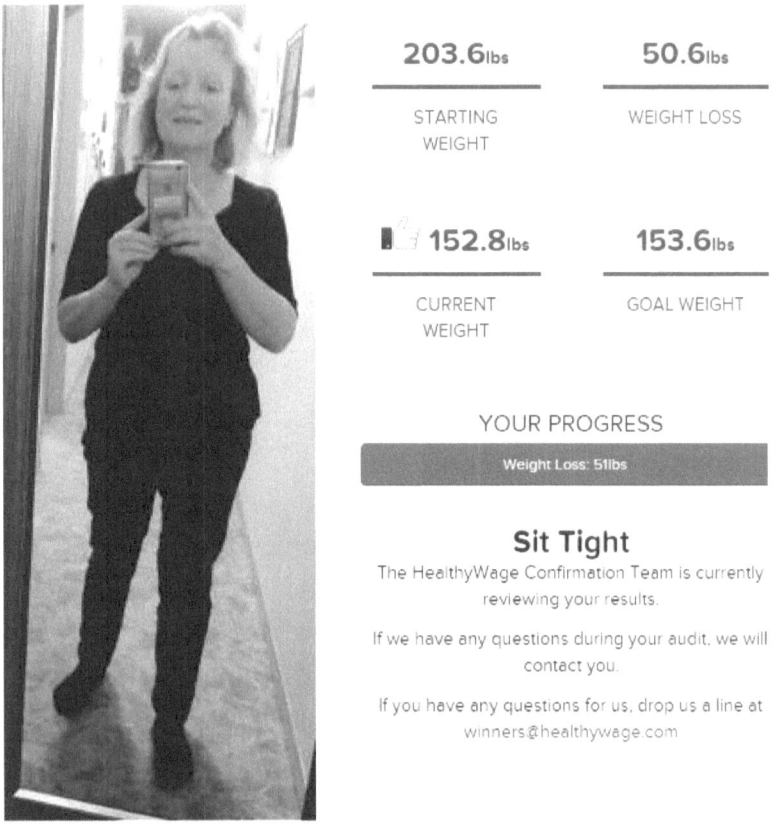

203.6lbs	50.6lbs
STARTING WEIGHT	WEIGHT LOSS
152.8lbs	153.6lbs
CURRENT WEIGHT	GOAL WEIGHT

YOUR PROGRESS

Weight Loss: 51lbs

Sit Tight

The HealthyWage Confirmation Team is currently reviewing your results.

If we have any questions during your audit, we will contact you.

If you have any questions for us, drop us a line at winners@healthywage.com

My healthy wage stats at right, and me today at my goal weight.

October 16, Friday

Weight: 154.1
Ate: Smoothies, oatmeal with cinnamon, coffee with Greens powder, and I can't remember what else. I broke my pattern and didn't write things down today.
Exercise: Dog walk: 16,465 steps

October 17, Saturday

Weight: 156.6
Ate: Smoothies, and I can't remember what else.
Exercise: Dog walk: 20,060 steps

Lesson Learned: Keep a Food Diary!

Today, I broke my pattern and didn't write down what I ate. And both today and yesterday, I didn't write in my diary. So of course I gained weight. Keeping track works! (Fortunately, I have the Fitbit to keep track of my steps for me, so I don't have to do anything but walk.)

October 18, Sunday

Weight: 158.3
Ate: 1 container Chocolate Obsession soy "ice cream," ½ bag of vegan chocolate chips, 1 box of vegan chocolate chip cookie mix (mostly raw), smoothie
Exercise: None to speak of: 4,144 steps

Vegan Pig-Out

I guess it's the "I might die tomorrow during surgery jitters," but I definitely found a way to pig out today, even though I am a vegan. Chocolate chips, cookie dough, soy ice cream…it all went down my soon-to-be-cut throat.

Of course, the sugar made me feel rotten, so I didn't get out of bed and walk the dogs all day. Stupid. Sugar really is a sick drug.

October 19, Monday

Weight: 159 at hospital (with clothes)
Ate: Pasta pesto, veggie burger, 2 small bowls of tomato soup, 3 cups of soy milk, 2 cups of juice
Exercise: Hospital walking: 7,485 steps (after surgery!)

Sent Home - Win!

Surgery went well…lasted about 3 hours. My neck is bandaged. I have about 5 to 10 pounds of fluids in me. Can't see my collarbones anymore. Miss them. I am trying to be the "good little patient" and lie still in my room, but to be honest, I just want to get up and walk and stretch and pop my poor back, which is far more painful than my cut throat since I can't sleep on most mattresses. So I do. I walk and walk and walk. I try to get Greg to bring a dog over to visit me. He doesn't. I walk some more. Down the hospital stairs, out the door to get some air, back down the halls.

My doctor, still here some 9 hours after my surgery, spots me, finds me back in my room. "Do you want to go home?" he quizzes me.

"Yes!" I say, gleefully, only regretting I just ordered pasta and a vegan burger from the menu since all I've had is tomato soup all day. *Starving!*

So I call Greg, and I go home. I'm a surgery success story, no doubt. I was 3 hours in surgery, lost half my thyroid and its lovely tumor (not sorry to see you go), and was supposed to spend the night in the hospital, being monitored and tested and poked, but instead I came home and slept with Kip hugging me, snoring softly and happily into my ear, and Miza growling a little because I love Kip so much. Harper slept on my feet, of course, and Blue slept on the couch next to my bed, watching me with love. All is good.

October 20, Tuesday

Weight: 164.8
Ate: 1 bag of cashews, ¼ cup of sunflower seeds, 2 smoothies, 1 roll with hummus, ½ cup vegan chocolate chips, oatmeal with chocolate protein powder and peanut butter
Exercise: None to speak of: 2,239 steps

Whoa! Post-Surgery Weight Gain!

It's gotta all be water weight, right? 5 to 10 pounds of water weight? Jesus!

Overall, today was rougher than yesterday with the great pain meds worn off. I stayed most of it in bed; managed to make two forms, but didn't get the poor ole dogs out on the trails.

October 21, Wednesday

Weight: 163.3
Ate: 2 smoothies, 1 Amy's frozen burrito, a chocolate pudding smoothie (avocado, frozen banana, chocolate powder, sunflower seeds, and peanut

butter)
Exercise: Dog walk: 11,051 steps
Still Fat

Hate being back in the 160s; I know I'll probably pee it off today. It's gotta be all those fluids in the hospital. I was bad (i.e., ate some vegan junk food, ate too much, didn't walk enough), but not that bad! Today, I'll go for a little dog walk, nothing strenuous until the throat cut has healed, but something beautiful anyway. Just waiting for Greg to get back from the gym and the sky to lighten a little.

Later: Had a beautiful walk by the river with the dogs. They were so joyous. I felt free and good; it was early enough that I didn't fear running into people. I haven't got to 10,000 steps since Saturday, but I'm going to try to get there today. Took off the outside bandage and see a long ugly scar, but not concerned. Love that I'm alive, survived, healthy, fit. Hoping to be back to the 150s soon! Tomorrow, perhaps?

October 22, Thursday

Weight: 161.3
Ate: 2 smoothies, 1 piece of seeded bread with hummus, 1 Amy's burrito, ¼ cup of sunflower seeds, 1 avocado, 3 carrots, 2 packages of nuts, 1 bowl of oatmeal with peanut butter and chocolate powder
Exercise: Dog walk: 7,130 steps

Recovering

The weight drops, about a pound a day, not the instant flush away of 10 pounds like I was hoping. This reminds me of how I hoped for an instant 50 pounds gone after having a baby, and then some elderly hospital volunteer telling me, "Don't worry, honey, he'll be out soon," as she looked at my colossal belly. It was almost a week after I'd given birth!

I still haven't gone to the – um – bathroom, so that will make a difference. It's been 5 days.

Anyway, I did make my 10,000 steps yesterday, managing the

last 2,500 by walking around the house, putting away things, reorganizing, cleaning. The dog walk was a 4,000-step shorter-than-usual one, but I was so happy to see my dogs run gleefully along the riverbank, happy to be out and free.

October 23, Friday

Weight: 156.3
Ate: 1 smoothie, 1 veggie/hummus wrap, ½ cup dark chocolate covered almonds, 1 Diet Pepsi, another smoothie with avocado, banana, sesame seed, oatmeal, carrots, and kale
Exercise: 2 dog walks and shopping: 20,790 steps!

Alive! And in the 150s Again!

Ah sigh. The weight falls back to the 150s – 5 pounds lost from yesterday, 8 pounds since the surgery gain. Wow, they must pump you full of fluids during surgery! Also, I was definitely plugged, and asked Greg to pick me up some ExLax at the store. The relief was instant. No reason to suffer...5 days without "going" was not comfortable.

I didn't panic; I didn't eat crazy, and most of all, I didn't stop eating or start starving. I didn't give up. I assumed it was fluids pumped into me during the surgery, and so it was.

Only made 5,000 steps yesterday; we tried to walk the hard Crevasse Moraine trails, but I was so cold and quite weak. I'm about to head out to some flatter, easier trails. I feel good; I am appreciating the rest period greatly. Surprisingly, I have had a lot of new form orders this week, but I've made them all, even the day after surgery. Mostly, I have played with, scratched, and talked to my dogs. I was even happy that my dear teenager talked with me yesterday...of course, he was lecturing me about quantum physics, and I let him enjoy the knowledge that he is smarter than I am in that area, as I know zilch. He didn't think it was funny when I offered to discuss poetry instead, but I did. Life is good; I'm happy; I'm alive!

October 24, Saturday

Weight: 155.3
Ate: 2 7-layer burritos (no sour cream or cheese); 1 vegan tortilla with veggies and hummus, 1 diet coke, 1 coffee with vanilla coconut creamer (not as good as it sounds),
Exercise: Dog walk: 11,416 steps

Baby E

My niece has the sweetest, cutest, most curious baby girl. She's 10 months old today. I love her so much. I was never a "baby person," except my own son, and now little E.

Little girl, little girl. Don't waste your days, months, years fretting about how you look, how much you weigh, what others think of your outside appearance. Find glory in the very fact that you are alive. Keep your spirit, sparkle, and happiness. Keep the innocence of childhood, and don't let others touch and maim your pure thoughts.

This is what I wish I could go back and teach little Jory, too.

October 25, Sunday

Weight: 157.3
Ate: 1 Italian meal and 1 appetizer at a restaurant – mostly eggplant and tomatoes. 1 Amy's burrito.
Exercise: Dog walk: 7,240 steps (went to Anchorage)

Sweet

Had a little fear last night; didn't sleep. My neck was swelling and painful; I thought the long surgery scary across my throat was going to burst, and I was going to die. So I stayed up all night watching *Sex in the City* reruns. Why not enjoy some NYC slut humor while dying? (And I use "slut" as a positive word. I've always liked it.)

Today, still alive, I went to lunch with Greg's family and a friend. I was so shocked and moved and touched by the kindness of one of Greg's family members, whom I haven't been all that nice to and have basically ignored for the last 15 years. She took my picture of me and Chewie on our last day together and had it printed and framed. She saw the same spirituality and love I saw in it. It sits next to my bed. Now why can't I be that thoughtful in gift giving? That will be a treasure to me the rest of my life! Here it is:

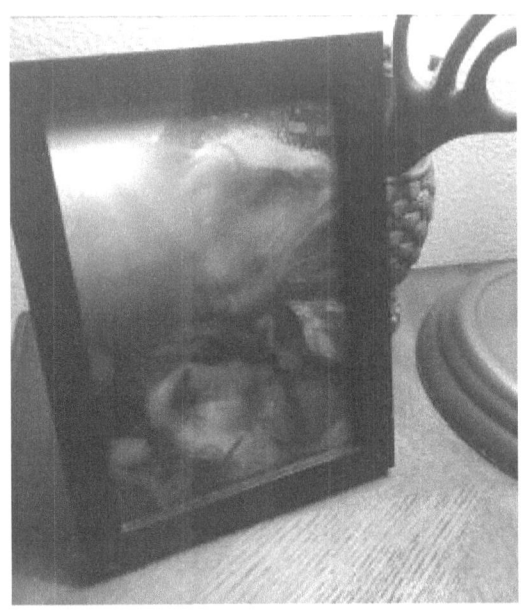

October 26, Monday

Weight: 157.4
Ate: 1 container of soy chocolate "ice cream" (1,040 calories); 1 Panini mushroom sandwich with chips
Exercise: 2 dog walks: 11,292 steps

Great Day

I feel really good, even if I did eat an entire carton of "ice cream" (not really…it's soy, all vegan!) today. Of course, I asked Greg to pick up the small one, but he brought home a large container, as it was all he could find. I had no discipline around ice cream, whether it's soy or not, so down it went. And felt good on my sore, scraped-thyroid swollen throat.

Also had a wonderful meeting with the board of directors of the organization I run…it's a nonprofit, all-volunteer, dedicated to saving the lives of animals by spaying and neutering, but I do almost all the work myself, so it was wonderful to get a new volunteer. Yay!

October 27, Tuesday

Weight: 157.4
Ate: 1 smoothie, 1 coffee with Greens powder, ¼ cup chocolate-covered almonds, ¼-cup roasted, salted hard corn, 1 veggie burger with Good Seed bread, 1 Amy's frozen lunch meal
Exercise: Dog walk: 13,768 steps

Back at TOPS

Missed last week at TOPS because of surgery recovery. It felt good to be back although I had to leave early because of work. Still, before throwing myself too much into my projects, I made myself walk the dogs and had a lovely time. It's amazing to be in Alaska in late October and have no snow and temperatures in the 40s. No one could be happier about this than me!

October 28, Wednesday

Weight: 155.8
Ate: Oatmeal, rye toast (1/2 slice), hash browns, 1 Amy's breakfast meal, 1 smoothie, ¼ cup raw pecans, ¼ cup corn nuts, ¼ cup vegan trail mix (no chocolate, or I would have eaten more!)
Exercise: 2 dog walks: 12,242 steps

Smoothies

My daily smoothies have helped me lose 55 pounds this year. You'd think people at my weight loss group would be curious what is in them. Instead they cringe at the color. Yes, it's a dark green/brown mixture, but so what? If you were in a weight-loss group, and one person was clearly excelling in her mission, wouldn't you be curious to know what works and why?

I try to tell them that the smoothies help me get in my fresh (and frozen) fruits and veggies every day, which is exceptional for a vegetarian who likes neither, as well as seeds or nuts. And of course I add a little cocoa powder or soy chocolate protein powder to put a chocolate zing in there. Perhaps the color is ugly, but the result is beautiful: my health, my weight loss, my success. I'm proud of me.

October 29, Thursday

Weight: 155.8
Ate: 2 smoothies, ¼ cup corn nuts, 1 large vegan cookie, 1 tortilla and veggie with hummus roll, ¼ cup trail mix
Exercise: Dog walk: 11,902 steps

And Another Size Bites the Dust... (a poem)

Another pair of pants falls off when I put them on.

Down another size.

Into the Goodwill bag.

Happy.

October 30, Friday

Weight: 155.1
Ate: 1 smoothie, ¼ cup salted baked corn,
Exercise: Dog walk: 16,448 steps

Cold Cometh...

So, we Alaskans have had a gloriously long, warm, unusual fall. Temps in the 40s for weeks and weeks. Happy long dog walks for me and my pack.

Today, the morning news team tells me cold weather has moved in. I'm about to set out for a walk in the 30s, dreading it, although I know much worse is to come. Even though I was born here, I'm not designed for cold weather. Brrrr. But dedicated dog owner (I prefer "companion") and weight-loss guru that I am, I'm outta here!

Later: It was actually seasonally warm, and snowflakes fell around us but didn't stick. We did a good, hard 10,000-step walk up and down trails. I amaze myself. I didn't even take one of Chewie's pain pills – hey, don't judge, it's the same thing they gave me in the hospital after my neck surgery but cost 10 times more since it was from vet: Tramodol. I have been astonished as it seems to be a pill that – although it doesn't make the fibromyalgia disappear – makes it bearable. Greg's noted how I've been walking faster and longer, and I said, it must be the pill. I hurt, but not as severe. I'm only taking 25 mg a day, but perhaps I've at last found a pill I can take that helps but doesn't make me feel drugged. We'll see. I'll wait for the follow-up with my thyroid doctor to see what he thinks.

October 31, Saturday

Weight: 155.1
Ate: Smoothie, vegan burrito, oatmeal with cinnamon, ½ cup dark chocolate covered almonds
Exercise: Dog walk: 11,797 steps

Two Years Ago…

I start to get confident about becoming Alaska State Queen for TOPS for this year (based on reaching goal by December 31; crowned next April), so I write a draft speech. I wanted to share it with you. Of course, it's planning for the future, but why not? Hasn't setting goals and planning for future success been part of my weight-loss journey all along? So here it is….

Two years ago, I attended the SRD weighing 240 pounds.

That was 100 pounds, 2 years, and a lifetime ago.

So much has changed since then.

Sometimes, change seems like the worst thing that could happen. I had a successful career as a technical editor and owned a forms business. Both made me rich. I could buy anything I wanted. But I didn't have time to enjoy anything. I spent at least 12 hours a day on the computer, 7 days a week. When I wasn't on the computer, I still had to check for orders on my phone. Every vacation was spent working. I had insomnia, anxiety, and money.

Now I am 100 pounds lighter, poorer, and happier. I don't fear getting fat again because I changed my way of eating completely.

It has been a long, hard road getting here, harder than writing a dissertation or than having my baby a few days shy of 40 years old.

That baby is about to turn 16 years old, and for almost 15 of those precious years I have fought, almost succeeded, and lost at trying to get to my pre-baby weight. Three times since joining TOPS, I have stood on this stage, a success story, going down, losing 25 or 50 pounds in the previous year. Three times I got to within 10 pounds of goal. Three times, I gained it all back, plus some.

I had all the perfect excuses. Here are some of them, in case you can relate to any and perhaps be inspired by what I was able to overcome. During that time I had several injuries and seven major surgeries. I live with chronic pain, the kind of pain that makes you want to cry or scream out loud sometimes, but you don't, because you were raised differently. I have spent well over $100,000 of my hard-earned dollars on surgeries and doctors. I have been prescribed and thrown away medication because although it helped with the pain, it caused weight gain, and I'd rather suffer than add more pounds. Can any of you relate?

I have spun into depression, thinking I would never lose weight. At the same time, I tried to quit smoking 300 times, and failed 299 of them, always gaining weight during the attempt until the last one, a year ago, during the middle of my weight loss journey. Plus, my thyroid had a tumor on it, which caused it to be sluggish. And then there's good ole DNA: When I was a child, I realized, upon seeing my relatives, that the women in my family tended to have the same shape as Alaska outhouses. So I'm genetically designed to be a 300-pound rectangle.

But finally, the reason I was fat all comes down to one word: *chocolate*. It's the only food I love; I never sickened of it; I craved it constantly. It made me happy; it made me high; it helped me through sad times and painful times. It helped keep me awake during many all-nighter editing sessions.

Fortunately, I love animals more than chocolate. I knew, this time, after the latest round of surgeries (neck, both shoulders, knee, and hysterectomy), when I got to my highest weight ever, that I had to go back to the only diet that ever worked or made sense for me: vegan. It allowed me to eat without counting calories, to eat without guilt, and to diet without dieting. It is a lifestyle change that is kind, easy, and it works. I knew this from a previous attempt at being vegan, but it was hard walking away from those Butterfingers and M&Ms again. Still, I did it.

This time, I did it for life. That way, I won't ever have to worry about being overweight again. And I can focus on other, more important things. It seems that, for women especially, our pursuit of the perfect figure (which will never happen, by the way), keeps us from living our lives, seeing old friends, believing in ourselves. That's sad.

So I gave up chocolate, but I only gave up milk chocolate. I still gift myself with the sweet sting of something chocolate every day. But mostly what I eat are fruits, vegetables, oatmeal, seeds, and nuts. Simple diet. Easy-peasy. It works for me.

Another thing I did was went to every single TOPS meeting I could, making TOPS a priority, and weigh-ins a necessity, even when I gained. I wish I had gone in those 2 weeks when I got to 240 pounds 2 years ago instead of hiding at home; then I would have a nice simple 100-pound weight loss recorded at TOPS, instead of 92 pounds weight loss. Don't be ashamed to go in and weigh in. It matters later, when you are losing, as you have more to be proud of!

And yes, I'm proud. I own this weight loss! I did it! Good for me! And good for you, all of you TOPS members, and I have met so many of you in the Valley and in Anchorage during my years there. You all patiently believed in me, and I appreciate that. I apologize for it taking me 15 years to "get it," but I've got it now. I want to say a special thank you to AK157, my first and last TOPS group, and to AK212, and AK13 during my time in Anchorage, for your incredible support, for making me laugh, for putting up with my odd sense of humor and my ADHD that makes me need to keep my hands busy, doing paperwork. You are awesome. I love you.

What I Did Right and Wrong This Month

What I have done right is:
- I walked my dogs, nearly every day.
- I made 10,000 steps most days, even after surgery (and 7,000 the day of surgery!)
- I stayed vegan.
- I ate healthy.
- I attended all TOPS meetings, except the one right after surgery.
- I didn't let surgery or pain bring me down or cause me to overeat, even when I gained nearly 10 pounds right after surgery (water weight).
- I made the healthywage.com goal (and received my check already!).
- I made it through a major candy holiday – Halloween – without candy.
- I lost weight.

What I have done wrong is:
- I'm still not a gym rat. I keep having to build myself up to this idea; I am so uncomfortable at gyms.
- That's it! I was awesome!

NOVEMBER

Weight: 155.5
Exercise Goal: 10,000 steps a day average, PLUS weight lifting at least 3 times per week
Inches: Chest: 42 Waist: 35.5 Hips: 41.75
Body Fat %: 27.45 BMI: 26-2/3
Motivation: To reach KOPS status at TOPS. Finally. After 14 years.

November 1, Sunday

Weight: 155.5
Ate: Rice toast (3 slices) with olive and black bean and garlic mixture, tomatoes, 2 smoothies, ½ cup dark chocolate covered almonds
Exercise: None (went to Anchorage): 6,045 steps

Inches and Percentages

For the first time my measurements and percentages increased across the board since I started this journey, mostly in fractions of an inch, but still. Hoping it's some residual water weight left over from the surgery. But I think I'm about done. Maybe 155 is all I can hope for, and I must be happy with it.

November 2, Monday

Weight: 155.8
Ate: Amy's breakfast meal,
Exercise: Dog walk: 10,048 steps

Snow

Well, it's here, inches of snow covering ice. The Friggin' Cold. Off to attempt a dog walk. Not excited. But a "must do." Based on my health, and the dogs' excitement. Wah.

November 3, Tuesday

Weight: 155.8
Ate: 1 cup hardened and salted corn, ½ cup dark chocolate covered almonds, 1 smoothie, 1 Amy's frozen dinner, 2 slices of rice bread with veggies, beans, and olives
Exercise: Dog walk: 12,358 steps

TOPS

Won the quarters. Not feeling the love at the TOPS meeting lately; maybe it's me, or maybe it's the envy of success. Certainly, I've been there. I know the feeling.

November 4, Wednesday

Weight: 156.4
Ate: ½ cup dark chocolate covered almonds, ½ cup vegan trail mix, 2 smoothies,
Exercise: Dog walk: 10,789 steps

Garbage

So I took my containers of salted hard corn and dark-chocolate covered almonds and tossed them in the garbage this morning. It was becoming out of control for me. The corn tasted like chips; the almonds like candy, and in a way they were, even if I did buy them in the "natural foods" section.

It's hard, I think, for many of us to throw out food. But I was either going to toss it in my body for added pounds, or toss it in the trash. I chose the trash. Proud of me.

Took my body out on the trails with the dogs and felt like I was going to freeze to death and die, and it's hardly winter yet, just dipping into the 20s. Maybe my fat layered me and kept me warmer. Or maybe I shouldn't have downed a smoothie just before the hike. In any case, I'm home now, warm, working, happy.

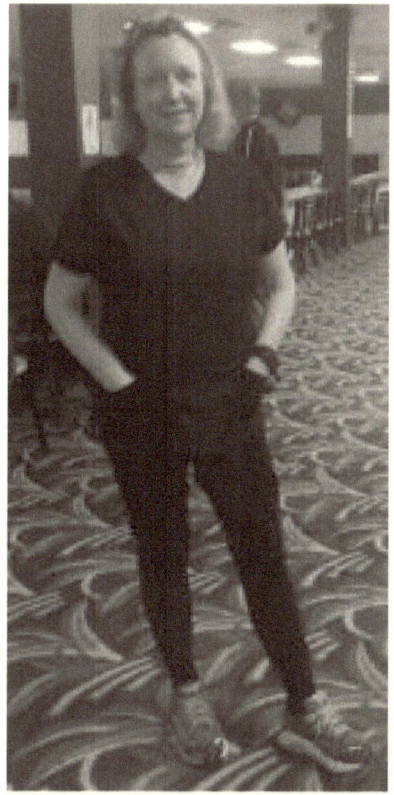

Neck still swollen from thyroid tumor removal surgery, but body is rocking!

November 5, Thursday

Weight: 156.8
Ate: 2 smoothies, black bean soup, 2 slices rice bread, ½ cup fried tofu and tomatoes, ¼ cup hummus, ½ cup seeds
Exercise: Dog walk: 13,149 steps

New Weight Goal

So I'm at the thyroid doctor follow-up appointment yesterday, and I ask him for a "prescription" for a goal weight for TOPS. I was going to say "155," because that's where I've been bouncing around the last almost 3 months. Seems to be where my body wants to settle.

Settle? I won't settle.

"148," I tell him.

He doesn't know how significant this is, but I walk out clinging that little scrap of paper, proud and confident and happy. I'm going to hit the 140s, even with the holidays coming up. I'm going to show others we can do this; we can not only not gain weight during November and December, but can lose it, achieve an awesome goal, break a plateau.

My son and Greg wail that I've somehow doomed the trip to Orlando I'll win for getting state queen at TOPS, but I just laugh at them. I'll make it.

I know I will.

Now I have a goal in mind – in hand, actually – and I'll get there.

November 6, Friday

Weight: 155.8
Ate: Garden burger with fries, 1 smoothie, 1 Amy's burrito, ¼ cup nuts, 1 handful of popcorn (offered the whole bucket, but declined – yay for my will power!)
Exercise: Dog walk: 10,452 steps

High Anxiety!

I'm sitting with Greg at a counselor's office this morning, for our first family counseling appointment. It had to be rescheduled for morning, so our son wasn't with us.

Which was probably a good thing.

What I envisioned for family counseling did not happen at all.

Let me put it this way: Greg was smiling and happy when we left while I was being sent to a psychiatrist for a referral, along with a request for expanding my Xanax prescription to "more."

"You are bouncing off the walls!" she said to me, after maybe 3 minutes.

"Thank you for understanding me," I said, sitting perfectly still in my chair (except for the standard body wiggling and hand wringing and leg swinging, perhaps, but those are my form of "normal"); however, my mind was bouncing like a giant rubber ball, per usual. "I was told it's ADHD."

"I don't think it's ADHD. Or rather, it could be ADHD, but it's something else too. I think it's extremely high anxiety. Are you like this all the time?"

"Yes, all the time," I said. "It's terrible," I added.

She's scribbling things, asking more questions, Greg is smiling as he knows he's got off easy (I'm certain he thought I was going to make it a Let's-Attack-Greg day, and I probably was).

Somehow, I feel strangely comforted. For the first time in my life, I believe a counselor "got me." And after only 3 minutes. Maybe I'll get help now. Maybe I'll get my worrying under control.

Maybe I'll breathe.

November 7, Saturday

Weight: 155.9
Ate: Smoothie, oatmeal with chocolate protein powder and peanut butter, 1 cup of soup
Exercise: Dog walk: 11,780 steps

Hawaii

My sister offers me her condo in Waikiki for a week. I say, "I can't handle the traveling alone right now." The truth is, I'm overwhelmed by the anxiety of traveling, fear of flying since 9/11, and the tasks of making reservations and finding taxis and such.

But Hawaii. Sigh.

My son won't miss a day of school. So he, my traveling companion since his birth, can't come. Maybe if Greg could come....

But there's the dogs....

It's all so hopeless, and yet I can't stop thinking of the sun, the beach, the ocean, the healing mentally and physically. The relaxing.

The only place I ever relaxed.

But I can't leave my son. Or my dogs.

After my teenage son is a complete asshole to me and his dad on the way home from bowling, I send a text to my niece, asking if she could consider staying here with the boy and the mutts, so Greg and I can have our first vacation together in 16 years.

She says yes!

I immediately text my sister, "Yes!"

I'm going to Hawaii.

And weight-wise, I have no doubt now that I will reach my goal, slim down, get stronger and fitter. Because beach-walking in Hawaii is the best exercise in the world for me.

Winning!

November 8, Sunday

Weight: 156
Ate: Smoothie, 1 cup of soup, ½ cup dark chocolate covered almonds, ½ cup seeds and nuts, 1 Amy's meal, 2 cups popcorn
Exercise: Dog walk: 12,492 steps

Thyroid

I'm hungry, I'm anxious, I'm in fibromyalgia pain. Interestingly, though, as I read online posts from people who've had partial or full thyroidectomies, as well as those on Synthroid (as I have been for years), I see numerous complaints about these problems. (Note: The frequent diagnoses of fibromyalgia surprised me, and made me hope the "cure" might be either in ending in the thyroid medication, which will take a couple months of tapering off, or in the removal of the tumor, which is done.). Of course, there's also those dreaded two words I don't want to read: *weight gain*. Nooooo!

I will battle it, as I always have.

Plus, I'm going to Hawaii. So I'll keep plugging away with my new way of eating, vegan and strong. Everything will work out fine; I believe this. Whether I'll actually reach the 140s by the end of year remains to be seen, but I believe in me. I will do my best.

November 9, Monday

Weight: 156.2
Ate: 2 smoothies, 1 hummus sandwich, ½ cup cashews
Exercise: Dog walk: 10,093 steps

Hunger

I suppose it's going to end up being one of those miserable days of hunger. Of course, I start my day feeling pretty good, with a deliciously healthy smoothie made of avocado, spinach, various fruits, and four types of seeds. Oh, and of course that little chocolate sting of happiness from the soy protein powder.

But tomorrow is the TOPS meeting and weigh-in, keeping me honest, and I'm a pound over a week ago. So that means a little less food today. Sigh. The weekly weigh-in is an awesome strategy, though, for someone like me. Preventing me from going too far up, especially when I have so many possible excuses (fibromyalgia pain, thyroid surgery, cold with winter here, anxiety, whatever…doesn't matter…it all comes down to eating too much and exercising too little causes weight gain, and I know this as well as anyone).

November 10, Tuesday

Weight: 155.6
Ate: 1.5 smoothies, 1 vegan cookie, 1 cup of popcorn, 1 cup of nuts, 1 Amy's breakfast meal, 1 bowl of oatmeal with protein powder and peanut butter
Exercise: Dog walk: 15,342 steps

Sigh

Dog walks are, for the first time in my life, just not a relaxing thing to do. I suppose it's the puppies that changed it all, although honestly they are sweet and loving and good. So perhaps it's the pack mentality. Mostly, I'm worried after reading a Facebook poster basically telling bikers how he sued a dog walker and made

20 grand from a dog attacking him on those same trails I use. I don't know how serious the attack was. My dogs have never bitten anyone, thank God, but that doesn't mean someone couldn't sue because they ran at them eagerly to say hello (as Blue did to a biker the other day). When did people stop saying hello to dogs? I always just say, "Hi there, doggie" in a kind happy voice, and that's that. We're pals. I'm not saying that always works, but it sure helps in most cases.

Lawsuits. I think, Geez, I could lose everything I worked too hard to earn because of stupid dog behavior. Then I think, maybe I could walk them separately, and a pack of four isn't running in front of me. But then I wonder, How will I find 4 hours in a day to walk dogs, and get anything else done? And how will I leave the others behind?

Through all my tragedies, losses, abusive relationship, breakups, tough times at jobs and schools…I had my pleasant, leashless, fun dog walks in the woods. It's kept me sane.

Now I wonder if I should anymore.

Later: Spent a wonderful evening cuddling with the dogs. Feel so much better. Ate too much. I seem to have a pattern of eating after I take my anxiety pill each evening. It seems to make me relax so much that I turn to food. Tonight that meant oatmeal (with peanut butter and chocolate protein powder) and nuts (cashews and almonds). Healthy foods, but still, not good for weight loss. Not sure how to handle the anxiety without the pill; not sure how to handle the pill without eating. Actions I need to take action on. I managed to get in over 15,000 steps today, in any case. Long dog walk, errands, shopping at a pet store with two dogs, then lots of housecleaning. And so it goes.

November 11, Wednesday

Weight: 157.2
Ate: oatmeal with cinnamon, 1 slice of dry rye toast, 1 small order of
hash browns, 1 Diet Pepsi, oatmeal with chocolate and peanut butter,

pita bread with garlic and hummus spreads, ½ cup nuts, 1 smoothie
Exercise: 10,595 steps

No Dog Walk

After yesterday, I dreaded the dog walk too much, the stress and worry of it. Plus we had freezing temperatures and the horrendous winds. So I stayed in. I did get my 10,000 steps. My house has never been so clean or organized as since I got a Fitbit! Great inspiration to keep moving.

November 12, Thursday

Weight: 158.1
Ate: Smoothie, Amy's meal, salad, ½ cup nuts, avocado, peanut butter, chocolate protein powder, hummus and herb crackers
Exercise: Short dog walk: 10,275 steps

I'm Off

Going to drive 10 miles to a place I can walk the dogs where I've only run into another person once. I should feel safer and happier there. There aren't any nice trails; we just stomp around the woods for a while, but I don't worry like I do on the well-used trails that my pack will get me in trouble.

Weight is going up, so I guess I need to hide the nuts (I'll put them in my packed suitcase for Hawaii!) and eat less. I know a lot of the consumption yesterday was salty, so that might account for some of it, but really that's just excuses. I'm hungry, and I need to do better. I was hoping the thyroid surgery would help with the hunger, but I guess this is just the way my body is, and I'll have to deal with it and accept it.

November 13, Friday

Weight: 157.5
Ate: Amy's burrito, vegetarian tamale, 1 cup of nuts, 1 smoothie, carrots, about 15 herb crackers
Exercise: Dog walk: 10,400 steps

Whole Foods

I find myself being drawn more and more to whole foods, especially fruits and vegetables. Although I have a freezer-full of Amy's vegan meals and burritos, I find myself turning away more and more from processed foods. I no longer buy things in boxes or cans. Yesterday, while grocery shopping, I found myself avoiding the frozen prepared meals. Instead, I bought fruits, vegetables, and a salad bag.

What is a salad bag? Well, it was the most delicious salad I ever had. In fact, it's the only delicious salad I ever had, to be honest. And it was easy for me, as everything was in the bag for me: greens, carrots, sesame sauce, flaxseed, and other goodies, all healthy and vegan. Had the irritating two servings in one package trick, so the calories are actually 200. How I hope my son learns to eat salads, long before I did in my mid-50s. The brand is "Fresh Express." Sadly, now that I've blown up the ingredients, I see it has sugar, so I guess it's not as healthy as I hoped. Ah me, it is so hard to be perfect when even the salad makers can't make it easy for me. Still, it gave me a healthy late-night snack, so I had an alternative to the usual high-calorie nuts and oatmeal plus peanut butter and chocolate onslaught.

As far as walks go, I bought another muzzle, this time for Harper Lee, so I can walk freely through the popular trails without worrying. (Except I'll still worry about Blue jumping happily toward a bicyclist, but she's so old and crippled, and just lost her sister, so I just don't want to put a muzzle on her.) Unfortunately, the temperatures have dipped into the single digits at night now. Hawaii. I just keep thinking Hawaii is coming. In 15 glorious days.

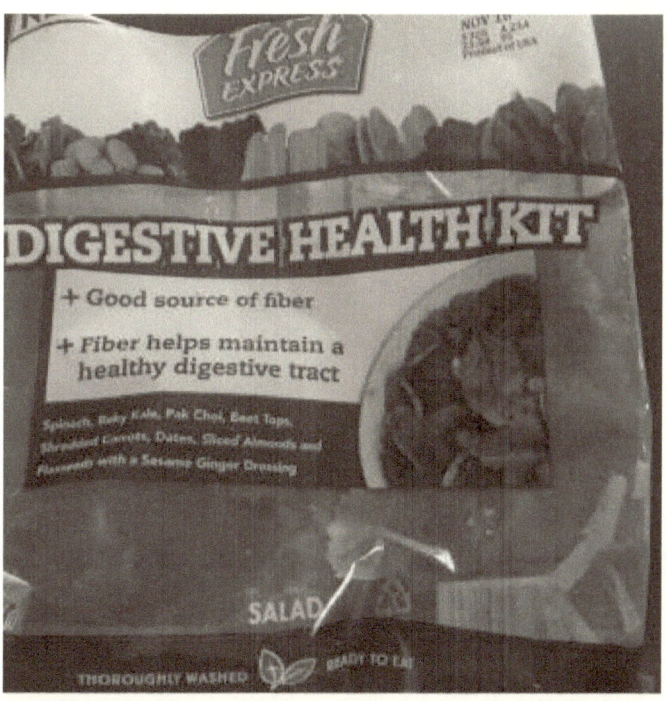

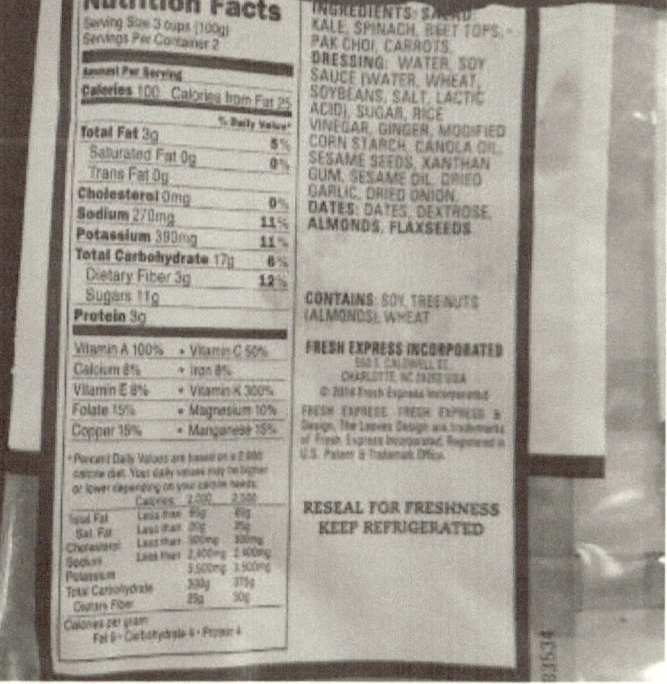

November 14, Saturday

Weight: 157
Ate: Smoothie, Amy's frozen dinner, 1 lollipop, 1 bowl of oatmeal with chocolate powder and peanut butter, 4 crackers
Exercise: 5,050 steps (too cold for a dog walk)

No, I Can't!

I can't dog walk today, dogs! I love you madly, desperately, fully. But I'm 1,000 years old and in pain and it's -2 degrees outside. Please don't make me. I'll play with you, dance with you, throw balls for you, cuddle you…we'll have fun. I promise. Inside. Where it's warm.

I peek ahead on the weather apps and see the temperatures are only getting worse for the next 4 days – dipping to 9 below zero. But then: next Thursday – right up into the roaring 20s! That sounds deliciously toasty right now. I'll take it. And, for an additional spin on positive thinking, I remind myself that in 5 weeks, the days will start "becoming longer," as we Alaskans like to say. Since summer solstice, darkness has stolen a little bit of every day, and for the next month, we spend much of our waking hours in eternal night. But then it turns around December 21, and a few minutes of light are added to each day. I think of that day as the beginning of spring hope. Of course, the worst and coldest months – January and February – lie ahead, but who's thinking that? Not me.

November 15, Sunday

Weight: 157.8
Ate: Smoothie, Amy's meal, about 2 cups of nuts and seeds (with salt), oatmeal with chocolate and peanut butter, Diet Coke (1/2 can), dark chocolate covered walnuts
Exercise: Dog walk: 5,607 steps
Inches: Chest: 42 Waist: 36 Hips: 42
Body Fat %: 27.55% BMI: 27

Stats Up

From my last measurements 2 weeks ago, my inches have gone up slightly, 0.5 inch in the waist, 0.25 in the hips. Not the direction I want to go. I'm more concerned that my BMI has gone up slightly; I want to get to the healthy range instead of the overweight category, so that is my goal now. (Plus I see in looking at my Excel data that my BMI is the same as it was 3 months ago…no real progress there.) My weight goal of 148 that I set out for myself with my doctor last week will bring me to a BMI under 25.8, so in the normal or healthy range. That is where I'm headed by the end of this year. It's going to take some work.

I've noticed since the thyroid surgery, and reduction of Synthroid, that I'm hungrier, and craving salt more. I have been adding lots of salt to my daily nuts and seeds, and I've been increasing the intake of those, particularly late at night. It's a learning process; I will have to teach my body how to function without the Synthroid while the thyroid hormones have to relearn to kick in without half a thyroid. Tricky! And most of all, I'll have to use my incredible will power to overcome the hunger. To top of it off, the cold weather has kept me from exercising as I should (and as my dogs need); we have about five more days of this, and then it will be in the 30s, if briefly, but enough time to give me some long, hard dog walks. That's the plan, anyway.

November 16, Monday

Weight: 158.4
Ate: Smoothie, 1 whole container of coconut milk "ice cream," Amy's burrito, dark chocolate covered walnuts
Exercise: Dog walk: 8,106 steps

Fun Times Ahead

Wasn't surprised by the weight increase because of all the salty nuts I consumed last night (finally tossing the last of them into the garbage), and the lack of real exercise (only about 5,000 steps a day the last 2 days, mostly just around the house). But getting too close to the 160s. Want to cry. But instead I'll walk, and semi-starve, and get back down. Losing weight was never supposed to be fun, right?

So when I say "semi-starve," I'm not kidding, really. I've been eating too much for my exercise output. Unless I want to exercise more (I don't, but I will in Hawaii for sure), I need to eat less. It will require some "suffering," I suppose, but I must remember that the hunger pangs won't kill me; it's temporary, and it's what works. I've proven I can maintain weight loss, within about a 5-pound range, pretty easily. Good. Good to know.

Now to lose the rest before the end of the year, and then maintain the rest of my life!

Alaska Winters and Hibernation

I have a sister who hates Alaska. She graduated from high school a year early, flew to Hawaii for college, moved to California later, and hardly ever came back, certainly not to live. While I shuddered through another short dog walk today (-3 degrees), and still am shivering an hour later, I think back to when I lived in the "states." I had my fat periods, usually when under incredible stress, overwork, and deadlines, but in general I was in much better shape there. Because there was no reason for winter hibernation. Walks did not get shorter in the winter. What Oregon and Washington consider "winter," we in Alaska call "August."

I think back to that same sister's theory she told me in high school. "In Alaska, we tend to be heavier because we need that fat layer to protect ourselves." As an example, she gave the blocky bodies of Eskimos, which at the point I hadn't seen many of, only paintings. She certainly didn't back it up with science. But it made some kind of odd sense, the idea that a layer of fat could actually be a life-saver from cold weather.

This comes to mind today because Greg has been looking at possible retirement property for us, somewhere warmer, perhaps inspired by my grumping that I can't stand winter here anymore, and after our son leaves for college, we're leaving too. This was a mantra I had for years, but the last two winters have been so mild and kind I've shut up about it till this week.

Greg found what looks to be a gorgeous 50 acres in rural Oregon. Hmmm. Tempting. Of course, I remember another side of rural Oregon, some bad things, and I won't go into them here. Instead, I'll just think of the 50 acres, my own personal dog park, winter temperatures in the 40s and 50s, which sounds like dreamland right now. But excuse me while I go hide under my blankets.

Dear Alaska, Part 1

Look, we've had a nice time. It's not you; it's me (okay, it's you). I thought we'd last forever, but the way you've turned so cold toward me lately, I'm going to have to let you go. I'm giving you 2 years' notice so you can find someone else, someone who appreciates you, who doesn't think long johns make her look fat, and who always remembers her mittens. (Plus my son doesn't graduate for 2 more years, so we can't divorce till then, Alaska.)

Stop crying, Alaska. We had it good while it lasted. Why can't you remember the fun times: June and July? Well, except in June you kept thinking it was funny to throw a thousand mosquitoes at my head. But we'll always have July, right? (And I'll pretend I don't remember the bear following me on the trails that one night; it never happened.)

So, thanks for the memories. I know I'll miss you and remember you fondly (once I finally get to escape you, that is). Except for November. And December. January and February were not good months for us, either, my love. But we'll always have July.

Love, Born-and-Raised-Here, so I didn't know any better.

November 17, Tuesday

Weight: 158.5

Ate: Smoothie, 1 (unfortunately large!) bag of trail mix, dark chocolate covered walnuts
Exercise: 3,944 steps (no dog walk; too cold)

Dear Alaska, Part 2

Dear Alaska,

Don't try to throw the northern lights in my face. You're always promising them, but every time I look they're not there.

I have been gentle and kind, but you don't fight fair. I feel your icy fingers at my throat even when I'm trying to sleep now.

Look, darling, I know I promised to stay with you "for better or for worse," but I had no idea you'd go this far down. "Feels like -21" today? Shame!

I trusted you. You gave me fireweeds and green leaves early these last 2 years, then caressed me with long summers and rainless, windless Alaska State Fair days!

I believed you that things would be different. That you had really changed. "I listened to Al Gore," you assured me, but it was all lies!

Dear love. I need a trial separation.

What? Well, yes, there's another.

His name is Hawaii. I'm sorry, but I can't resist his charms. I'll be back soon, and I hope you're nicer to me upon my return.

Dear Jory:

You are going to HAWAII?! You cheating, lying, ignorant slut! How can you forget I gave you this?

FU, Alaska

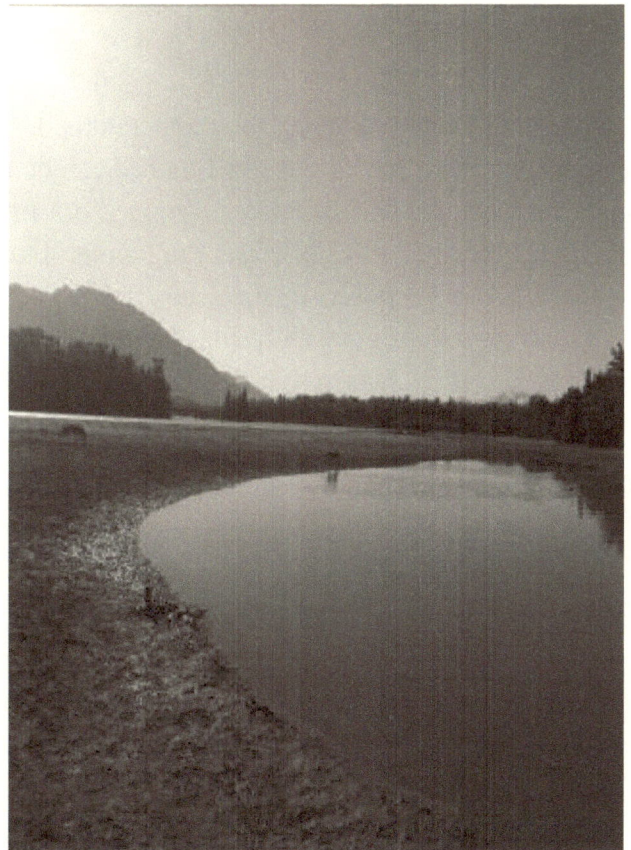

Dear Alaska,

In response to your last post ("FU"? Really? After all I've endured from you?), I want to forgive and forget. But my friend Shelley reminded me that I was not your one and only woman that you slammed down on the ice numerous times, sending me for knee and shoulder repairs. So maybe it is I who should be saying FU. But I just can't forget what you did for me in July. So I forgive you.

November 18, Wednesday

Weight: 159.0
Ate: Amy's burrito, stir fried vegetables, 3 dark chocolate covered almonds, oatmeal with peanut butter and chocolate protein powder, ¼ cup seeds, ½ box of Special K with almonds cereal (dry)

Exercise: 6,755 steps (no dog walk; too cold)

Gaining

So I'm gaining this week since the temperatures have stayed below freezing, and what few dog walks I've had can be measured in 10-minute increments. The steps have dropped drastically. I'm eating too much for the little exercise I'm doing. Excited that tomorrow the 30s are supposed to magically reappear, which is nice since the last few days have all been subzero: -21 yesterday, -17 today. Yuck! Escaping Alaska sounds so nice right now.

Therapy, SSRIs, and Weight Gain

Had a family counseling session last night, then the first appointment with the psychiatrist this morning. Took Greg. Refused to step on the scale. "It looks like a cattle scale," I whispered to Greg, and he said it's probably for wheelchairs. Something about it, and weighing in front of Greg after my 5-pound gain this week, plus having layered myself with numerous clothes and jeans and heavy shirts, sounded awful. I knew I'd see the 160s again, and it wouldn't be fair or right.

The session focused on my anxiety and worrying. The answer, according to the psychiatrist, is that he wants to try me on Zoloft, a very small amount (25 mg), which we'll need to increase till we find the "right" dose, but it sounds like that will take forever and a day, since it takes 3 weeks to feel any effects. But of course, I only had one real concern.

"Will it cause weight gain?" I wanted to know.

Always myself.

"No," he assured me, scratching something in my chart. But when I look it up later, I see most of the SSRIs do tend to cause weight gain. I want to cry. Should I take it or not? One site says: "Like many other antidepressants, use of Zoloft has been associated with weight gain."

Wellbutrin seems to be the only antidepressant that doesn't

cause weight gain, in fact, can help with loss, but he didn't want me on that one. It's more for the anxiety than the depression.

What to do…what to do?

Crap. I really do hate drugs.

November 19, Thursday

Weight: 159.8
Ate: Smoothie; salad with peas, sesame seeds and sauce, apples, and avocado; Amy's dinner, about 1 cup of roasted sesame seeds
Exercise: Dog walk: 10,738 steps

More Weight Gain

So close to the 160s again. Fortunately, the weather has warmed up to above freezing (9 degrees, wow), so I'm about to embark on a dog-walking adventure. Sitting inside the last few days has not been good for my weight, that's for sure. I'm also hungrier than ever, which might be because of the reduction of Synthroid. And on top of that, the anxiety medication takes away my ability to control my hunger, so I snack more (last night's cereal and seeds, for example).

I am working on finding balance. I had my blood drawn to check my thyroid levels, and I'm seeing a counselor now, which I guess is good. So far the suggestions seem to steer toward medication, but I'm hoping there will be other insights as we go on.

November 20, Friday

Weight: 159.3
Ate: Smoothies, salad, soup, Amy's frozen meal, nuts and seeds
Exercise: Dog walk: 10,237 steps

Salad

Yesterday, I made a salad. Well, I bought a kit, which just had sesame sauce and pea pods, but then I cut up apples and avocado, roasted some raw sesame seeds, and mixed it all together. Used it throughout the day and night for snacking.

This seems like a simple thing to you, probably a normal person, but for me, who (a) doesn't like salad, (b) used to hate vegetables (even though a vegetarian), and (c) avoids cooking or preparing her own food, it was huge. And a sign of good things to come. And I lost 0.6 pounds and didn't go hungry because when I wanted a snack, especially late at night, I grabbed my big bowl of premade salad. Healthy win. Much better than the nuts or peanut butter and chocolate oatmeal I usually eat at night.

November 21, Saturday

Weight: 158.3
Ate: Smoothie, salad, stir fry veggies
Exercise: Gym: 8,626 steps

Salads and Gym

Went to the gym today and worked out, plus stuck to salads and stir-fry veggies for food. Trying to contain the gain.

November 22, Sunday

Weight: 159.9
Ate: Smoothie, salad, coffee with plant powder, stir fry veggies
Exercise: 5,306 steps

Unfair

Life is not fair. Yesterday I lived on salads and veggies, and still I gained over a pound. I'm pretty certain this has something to do with either (1) the weaning off the Synthroid (down to half a tablet a day), or (2) the prescription for an antidepressant (for anxiety). I am not coming this far without reaching goal. I could not be hungrier, by the way.

Later: I can't believe the Walgreens pharmacy actually called me to see how I'm doing on the Zoloft. I said I was gaining weight and not happy about that.

She said since it's for anxiety she likes Paxil and Lexapro – if the doctor wants me on an SSRI. But she agrees with my pharmacist friend hat Buspar is a great one for anxiety/worrying, since depression isn't really an issue, and it doesn't cause weight gain like the SSRIs. I'm going to check with the psychiatrist tomorrow about switching to Buspar.

Of course I've worked and starved to lose 85 pounds and do not want to gain one pound back; I've already gained several pounds since starting!

November 23, Monday

Weight: 157.6
Ate: Salad, 2 smoothies, stir fry veggies
Exercise: 2 dog walks: 10,687 steps

Down 2 pounds, but this woman can't live on salads and smoothies forever! At least I hope I don't have to!

Yahoo! Health's Weight-Loss Win Series

It's been a while since I've posted book, movie, or Internet reviews, so I wanted to bring up a site that is inspiring: Weight-Loss Win, authored by Andie Mitchell, which tells the stories of people who have lost from 40 to well over 100 pounds. In short, simple stories they explain their diet dramas, and how they claimed victory. Sometimes, it's attitude, as in Shannon Robinson's post, wherein she describes losing 59 pounds. She writes:

> *I've learned to love myself from every angle and at every stage. I've gained confidence and joy and drive. I have a passion for life and for learning and for becoming the best possible version of myself. For me, it isn't about the pounds. I actually haven't gotten on the scale in two months. The scale can drive a girl insane! I want to be stronger, faster, and better than I was yesterday. That's it. No more "just five more pounds and I'll be happy," or, "If I could just have a little more definition in my stomach, I'll be happy." I am happy NOW – at this weight, at this pants size, at this stage in my journey and in my life. I am happy.*

This makes me think how nice it will be not to have to weigh myself daily or worry about the number on the scale. I still hope to get into the 140s before being "done," because I know it will be healthier and I feel fittest when I don't have fat around my back and belly. But whatever my body tells me…I'll stop there.

I find these stories interesting, inspiring, useful, and perhaps you will do. Especially if you're locked inside on a cold, winter day but trying to avoid the refrigerator.

November 24, Tuesday

Weight: 157.5
Ate: 2 smoothies, 1 vegan waffle, then forgot to write down my foods
Exercise: Dog walk: 7,015 steps

Freedom

TOPS and schools were cancelled today because of slick roads. This somehow gave me the freedom, after making my son waffles for breakfast, to make my own vegan ones, which I've never tried. Since they were sugarless, and he'd downed all the syrup, I can't say they were that great. But the dogs enjoyed the leftovers, anyway. (And it does remind me how important that weekly weigh-in is to keep me honest and dedicated.)

I spent the last 2 days on smoothies and salads. I supposed, if I have to, I can live like that, but it's a little too simplistic, even for me. I need *some* variety. Also, the rewards weren't worth the starvation…down 2 pounds in one day, but none the next. I know little of this has to do with me; I am on half the Synthroid now, plus an antidepressant for the anxiety. God knows what is going on with my body's metabolism.

November 26, Thursday

Weight: Did not weigh (159.7 yesterday)
Ate: Sweet potato and veggies dish, 1 roll, noodles and veggies dish (3 helpings)
Exercise: Dog walk: 5,688 steps

A Break

I didn't want to weigh myself today, so I didn't. It's the first time in this weight-loss journey (except when I was in a hotel and couldn't), where I didn't. It was too much. I know I'm gaining, and I know it's Thanksgiving. I am thankful for discovering my health this year, and for losing so much weight. I want to focus on that, not the gain, today. (Yesterday, although I know I did 12,061 steps thanks to the Fitbit, and I ate the typical burrito, smoothie, vegan cookie, and veggies, I did not write in my journal. I wonder if the winter is getting to me? It's not like me to avoid writing.)

November 27, Friday

Weight: 161.9
Ate: Smoothie, ¼ cup seeds, ½ cup dark chocolate covered almonds, 1 large order of French fries
Exercise: Dog walk: 11,357 steps

160s...sigh

So here's the deal. I see the weight gain. I don't blame myself. I blame the thyroid not kicking in yet, to compensate for reducing the Synthroid, and I blame the antidepressant, which is an SSRI, and causes weight gain (or "can cause weight gain," which for me always means, "you'll get fat").

November 28, Saturday

Weight: 161.9
Ate: Smoothie, Amy's meal, seeds, nuts, fruit
Exercise: 16,322 steps (even though I was on an airplane most of the day)

Hawaii

I'm taking a week-long break from recording what I eat, but I've packed my soups and vitamins and seeds. I'm about to embark on a great healthy week of beach walking in the warm sun. It will be my first vacation without my son since he was born. It will also be my first vacation with his dad since my son was born. Just us.

Wish me luck. I'll see you thinner! And tanner! Until December 8, then!

What I Did Right and Wrong This Month

What I have done right is:

- Stayed vegan.
- Exercised every day.
- Never binged.
- Pursued improving my mental health (anxiety) by seeking counseling.

What I have done wrong is:

- Nothing. I didn't lose weight, though.

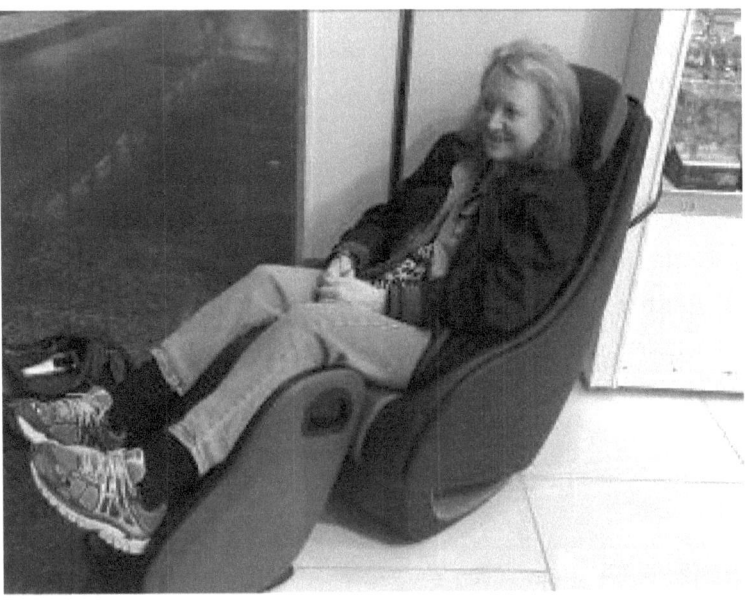

At the airport on the way to Hawaii; massage chair felt great! (And I fit in it!)

DECEMBER

Weight: 156.4 (December 8)
Inches: Chest: 40.5 Waist: 35 Hips: 40.5
Body Fat %: 27.20 BMI: 26-5/6
Motivation: To be TOPS Queen. To reach goal. To be healthy and strong and fit. To live long and prosper (hello, Spock!)

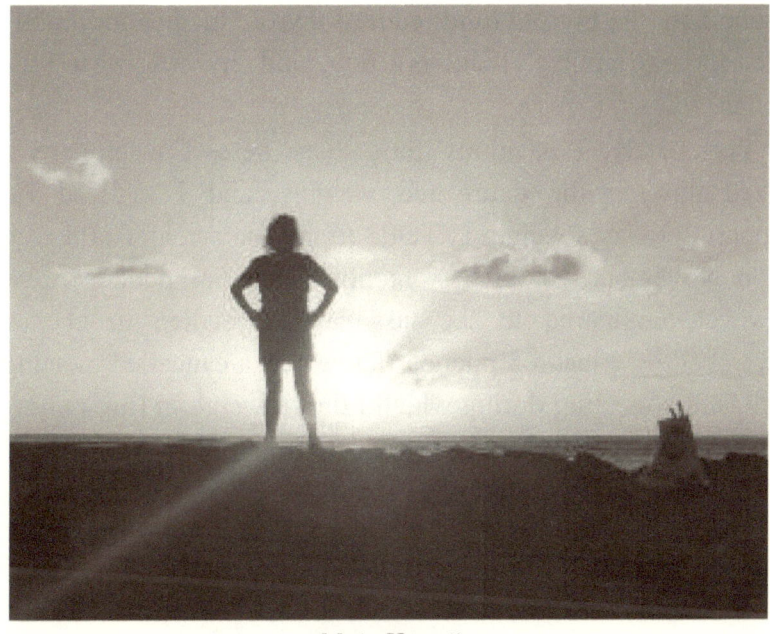

Me in Hawaii

December 8, Tuesday

Weight: 156.4
Ate: ¼ cup popcorn, smoothie
Exercise: 4,891 steps (plus two short dog walks; forgot the Fitbit)

Back from Hawaii

I worked hard, over 30,000 steps a day (I'm not kidding – screenshot below), and I ate sparingly, mostly my vegan soups and seeds I brought with me. I sand-walked. I even walked from Waikiki to the top of Diamond Head crater and back down again (38,000 steps that day). The only local food I ate was fresh fruit whipped in a bowl to the texture of ice cream, with granola and fruit bits, but I ended up with a great case (my first) of "traveler's diarrhea," which is just as fun as it sounds.

And I gained weight. Totally unfair. Really, really wrong.

I did lose inches, so I'm happy for that. But I know there is absolutely no reason I shouldn't have lost 10 pounds as hard as I worked and as little as I ate, so I can only blame my incredible metabolism, the thyroid (and reduced thyroid medication), and the SSRI for my anxiety. I did my best, and my best wasn't good enough.

Fortunately, I have my food diary here. I went back and looked through the dates and weights, and I realized I am comparing today's weight at TOPS to the last actual TOPS weigh-in on November 10: after a month, I am 0.4 pounds heavier. However, compared to the last day I weighed in at home, November 28, I lost 5.5 pounds. There was a cancelled meeting in there, and a meeting during which I didn't weigh in (my only time doing that for the year).

So, deep breath, I'm doing okay.

Nov 29 – Dec 5, 2015		220,058 steps	
12/5	**25,509** steps	★	>
12/4	**20,802** steps	★	>
12/3	**32,745** steps	★	>
12/2	**35,667** steps	★	>
12/1	**35,590** steps	★	>
11/30	**38,168** steps	★	>
11/29	**31,577** steps	★	>
Nov 22 – 28, 2015		68,436 steps	

December 9, Wednesday

Weight: 156.5
Ate: Smoothie, Amy's burrito, ¾ cup almonds, one 8-inch vegan pizza,
tofurky, banana, grapes
Exercise: Dog walk: 8,680 steps

Done with Zoloft

So I saw my counselor. I'm done with the Zoloft. I haven't
seen any change in my anxiety levels to compensate for what
seems to be a (potential?) increase in weight, or more difficulty
losing. So I'm done. Whether or not I'll try something else I'm not
sure. I know I "self-medicated" my anxiety in the past by eating
milk chocolate and smoking cigarettes, and now those two items
are off the table. I am still chewing nicotine gum, but I'm thinking
that is actually making the anxiety worse. So I suppose it is time to
let go of that as well. Goodbye to nicotine forever. Whatever
purpose you served me, I'm done with you.

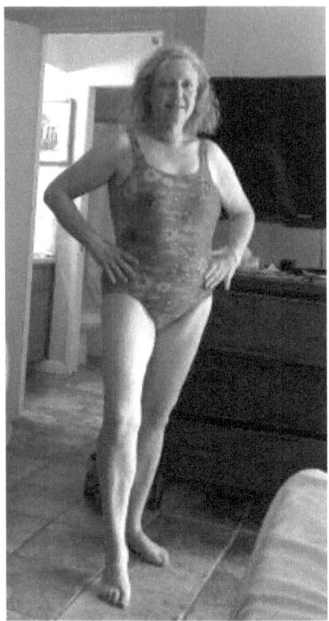

Yes, I dared to have a swimsuit picture of me taken in Hawaii. Crazy! Been uncountable years since I let that happen.

December 10, Thursday

Weight: 155.1
Ate: Smoothie, tofurky, 2 cups popcorn, hummus and chips, carrots, Amy's meal
Exercise: Dog walk: 8,678 steps

Final Weight Goal?

Is the body in a plateau, or is the body at the finish line?

I'm not sure. It's up to my body. I feed it good nutrition; I take care of it by giving it daily exercise (walking). I could do more, work out harder, like I did in Hawaii, where I saw inches drop, if not pounds. But I don't want to spend my days working full time on my body. An hour or so of dog walking is good enough for me.

I feel good at 155. There's a little more "poof" I'd love to drop around my back and belly, but mostly at this point, honestly, it's skin. Yes, sadly, this time I don't just have excess skin in the neck, but also in the stomach and under the arms. The joy of gaining nearly 100 pounds and then losing most of it when you're over 50,

I suppose. It doesn't matter…I look good, feel good, feel stronger, fitter, and healthier. And isn't that what it's about? As the last 2 weeks of 2015 come closer, I realize that I've reached my goal, and I'm at peace. Whatever the final number is, that is my number. I will claim it for my KOPS status at TOPS. I have the "doctor's prescription": anywhere from 148 to 155. I'm here. I've landed. Whew!

December 11, Friday

Weight: 155.5
Ate: Smoothie, Amy's burrito, nuts, seeds, carrots, hummus and chips, popcorn, soy Chocolate Obsession "ice cream" (1 pint), dark chocolate covered almonds
Exercise: 10,837 steps

The Abuser

I look up the abuser. He's a person I dated in Oregon, on and off, for 7 years. Every once in a while I check to see if he's dead or married or in jail for murdering a woman or what. I don't know why. I just do.

A photo finally shows up on the Internet. He's friggin' gorgeous still, more beautiful than ever. I hate that. I wanted his outside to reflect every time he hit me and hit other women. Nope. His muscles ripple. He's tan and hot and his blond hair has grayed to a devastatingly handsome shade.

Life is unfair. Fortunately, I am not bad looking myself, for a 55-year-old lady. Maybe someday he'll look me up and be sorry. Probably not.

December 12, Saturday

Weight: 156
Ate: 1.5 large popcorns, no butter, at the movies. ½ cup almonds. ½ cup sesame sticks. ½ vegan wrap with veggies. ¼ pear, dark chocolate covered almonds
Exercise: 4,890 steps

The Hunger Games

Went to the final *Hunger* Games movie with the family. Glad that's over. Okay, okay. I'm sorry, *Hunger Games* fans. I remember, as excited as I was that my son was reading a book, way back in fourth grade, I was a bit shocked when he told me the plot. All I could think of was the coliseum. With children! Yuck!

It's weird that I'm playing the Hunger Games too, as in, I'm hungry. Much hungrier than I was in Hawaii, although I am eating ten times as much. Today I ate no meals but munched "healthy" snacks (except really, a giant butterless movie popcorn cannot be called healthy by any stretch of the imagination). I went to bed most of the day; the *Hunger Games* depressed me thoroughly, and unfortunately, we went to the early show. My day was done. My lovely dogs went walkless, but it being Saturday, the trails full, and yesterday's fiasco of Harper chasing some poor dog around a park, frightening it, drove me to bed. I shall have to walk these dang pups separately until they learn some manners, if they ever do. Fortunately, they cuddled and loved me all afternoon, happy to just be with me.

December 13, Sunday

Weight: 156.5
Ate: Amy's meal, oatmeal, smoothie, hummus and chips, banana
Exercise: Dog walk: 10,569 steps

The Little SSRI Pill

So I dropped out of the SSRI pills (Zoloft) Wednesday through Saturday. I gained a pound. I took one this morning. I don't know what to do about my mental or physical state. I'm confused. I know I don't want to gain weight. That's one thing I know for sure. I do think back on Hawaii, and how little I ate, yet how much I walked, and I think, I really wasn't that hungry. Maybe the little pill helped? I have no idea. I decide to give it another try, but this time taking the full prescription of the

Synthroid. One of them is affecting my weight; perhaps it's the thyroid medication.

Another thing is that I'm not exercising. My steps plummeted from 35,000 a day (at least 15 miles daily!) in Hawaii to barely 5,000 a day since I got home to Alaska. The fibromyalgia pain, gone in the warm weather, is back full force. The dark and cold throw me into depression. My fear of the puppies' trail behavior wears me out. Overall, I'm unhappy. I spend most of my time in bed, when I'm not working.

December 14, Monday

Weight: 156.7
Ate: Amy's burrito, smoothie, 2 cups almonds, ¼ cup corn nuts, 1 vegan wrap with beans and veggies
Exercise: Dog walk: 15,485 steps

Fear Aggression and Littermate Syndrome

I should title this one "solutions" because today I took action on Kip's fear aggression. Why are dog issues a part of my weight loss book? Because first of all, I have lost 70 pounds since I took in those foster puppies a year ago last October. Some of that is due to them: walking them, cleaning up after them. Most of all, feeling loved by them. Being adored by them.

Second of all, as you well know, I am having issues with the puppies, in particular Kip, with his fear aggression toward other dogs. It has increased my anxiety level to the extreme. It has taken the joy out of dog walks, for the first time in my life.

So today, coming back from the trails, watching off-leash dogs running gleefully toward my leashed insane puppies, and the fearful owners grabbing their dogs and glaring at me in the typical "shame on you" look of horror, I took an action I never thought I'd do. I went home and searched online for a trainer that boards. I called them, explained the problem, took both puppies there, stayed for hours, and left them with a $1,250 check and Kip. For 2 weeks.

In the meantime, I will work with Harper without her brother. Turns out they have "littermate syndrome," which actually is a "thing." I was lucky Blue and Chewie didn't have it. But Kip and Harper definitely do. Harper, it turns out, is the leader. Kip hides behind her and me. He is going to learn to be confident, to stand on his own, to not get me in trouble for the next 12 years or so of his life. At least that's the plan.

I go back in a week to work with him. I feel bad, but I also feel good. Hope. I definitely miss my "baby," and crave his cuddles and sighs, but we're going to make it through this. Better. I dedicate the next 2 weeks to learning everything I can to help my puppies become better, safer, more secure dogs.

December 15, Tuesday

Weight: 156
Ate: 2 vegan burritos, 1 cup sunflower seeds, 1 smoothie, ½ cup chocolate covered almonds, 1 vegan wrap with beans and veggies
Exercise: Dog walk: 9,592 steps

Home Again

Kip came home again. He "faked" being sick so the trainer called me. I'm happy; Kip's happy; we're snuggling tonight. I take him back Thursday. Here is his expression on getting to come home from "school" early; note the tail wag:

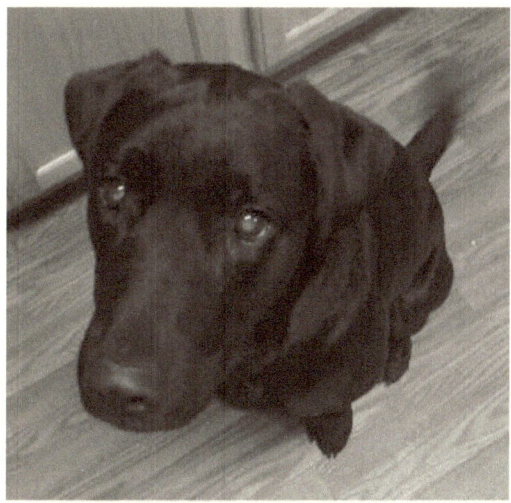

My beloved Kip.

December 16, Wednesday

Weight: 155.8
Ate: 2 vegan burritos, 1 cup sunflower seeds, 1 smoothie, ½ cup chocolate covered almonds
Exercise: Dog walk: 11,188 steps

TOPS

At TOPS yesterday, they asked me if I've reached my goal. I said, "I guess so. Hawaii was a test to see if I'm plateaued or actually done, and it appears that my body is done. I could not have worked out harder or ate less for those 7 days."

My Fitbit friends agreed; they'd seen my 35,000 steps and 15- to 16-mile days, live, as it happened, on their own phones.

So I said, "Whatever weight I am the last Tuesday of the month, in 2 weeks, that's it, I'm done. I have doctor's prescriptions anywhere from 148 to 155, so I'm good."

"What if the last day there is a storm, and TOPS is cancelled?" Marguerite asked.

We all looked at her. That would mean I would be ineligible to win 2015 "queen" and the Orlando trip in July. That means I'd have to wait till next year to be a KOPS. Good thinking.

"So, I guess I'm done next Tuesday," I said. So December 22, I will reach my TOPS goal. Whatever it shall be.

December 17, Thursday

Weight: 155.7
Ate: 2 vegan burritos, 1 cup sunflower seeds, ½ cup chocolate covered almonds
Exercise: Dog walk: 10,892 steps

Walk-about

Just came back from a dog walk. With three dogs and no Greg. It was pretty peaceful. Harper stayed close. Kip is back at the trainer's. No one was in the parking lot when I left although it was filling up with cars by the time I returned. I liked being out in the wild of Alaska alone with my dogs again. That's how it should be; how I'm most comfortable. Not to say there's anything wrong with Greg – he's awesome to come along. But it's a "have to" have him because of Kip thing. We both know it is.

God bless my beloved Kip, and I hope and pray the trainer helps him. If not, he may forever have to be walked on a leash, alone.

December 18, Friday

Weight: 156
Ate: Smoothie, avocado, Amy's burrito, ½ cup nuts, ½ cup seeds, 1 cup sesame seed snack crackers
Exercise: 10,152 steps

5 Days

Five days till the KOPS weigh-in; four days of dieting and exercise ahead. I'd really like it to be an "even number" loss for my highest TOPS weigh in, which would be 80 pounds if I get to 152. (I actually weighed 8 pounds more last year, my highest at 240, but I didn't go in to the meetings those 2 weeks as I was so ashamed!) I don't seem to do well with "even numbers" though, so I have my doubts. Plus I'm hungry. And so it goes. I'll just do my best!

December 19, Saturday

Weight: 154.1
Ate: 2 smoothies, 1 cup of olives with olive oil, 1 small Diet Coke, 1 piece of celery, ¼ cup of seeds, 2 cups of popcorn
Exercise: 10,240 steps

Weight Loss

Nice how I lost two pounds in a day without trying. In fact, I didn't go for a dog walk yesterday. I had to do my last 6,000 steps just walking around the house late last night. I spent almost all of yesterday editing a report for a rush job. But I made it to 10,000 steps even so.

I appreciated the work distraction from my obsessive anxiety over worrying about Kip, missing Kip, wondering about Kip...oh my God! It's driving me mad! I miss that little bugger. I hope training is going well. I realize that much of my ability to lose weight this year and quit smoking are due to the love and adoration from my puppies; they calm me. Unfortunately, they also give me anxiety when they behave badly around other dogs.

December 20, Sunday

Weight: 156.7
Ate: 1 Amy's burrito, 1 smoothie, 1 cup dark chocolate-covered almonds
Exercise: 7,559 steps

Some Dream

I must have had some dream. I gained almost 3 pounds! Ha! I'm sure it will come right off; probably due to the salty popcorn I ate last night. But amazing how fast I can gain weight. Geez.

Mostly my issue is anxiety from missing Kip, worrying about Kip, wondering about my little scared pup. Day 4; 12 to go.

December 21 – December 24

Weight: 154

Exercise: Averaged 10,200 steps

KOPS, So What?

So I made/claimed KOPS on Tuesday, December 22, but I am deep in anxiety and depression. I thought seeing Kip at the trainer's yesterday would help, but it made it a thousand times worse. He is starving to death, literally, since he won't eat; he's terrified. Oh, how he tried to run and run to run to me, to run away from the trainer. How he kept getting flipped over by the trainer jerking on his leash. How I wanted to scream and grab him and run away with my poor baby dog. (I would have, but my counseling made me promise to take a Xanax before I went out there; she looked up what kind of trainer he was ["balanced" – don't use them I learned later; use positive reinforcement; they also don't make you leave your dog with them – I didn't learn this till later] and knew it would be bad. The trainer wouldn't even let me say hi to Kip or hug him or acknowledge him. What the F? He's been using a shock collar on him and only feeding for "rewards" (looks like Kip hasn't earned any). How terrified my puppy was. How finally I was "allowed" to feed him treats and how happy he was at last to be next to me. How he ran away after we left, looking for me, so we drove back; he came to me from the woods; I took him back to the trainer's and left him. Every pore of me wanted to bring him home; I was screaming inside and still am. It was awful. I have till next Tuesday at 12:30; they will bring him over then. I can't stand it. I want to die. I feel so terrible for my little Kippers. I love him so much. He is so wretched and frightened and miserable. He is so scared. Most everyone tells me to leave him there; a scared dog is a dangerous dog; an insecure dog is bad news; whatever. All I know is I love him and he loves me and I can't bear it. And I don't care a crap about anything else right now. I made KOPS. Whoopie. Fuck.

December 25-31

Weight: 153.3
Exercise: Averaged about 7,200 steps

End of the Year

So I made it to the end of the year with a 57-pound weight loss for the year, and a total of 87 pounds since my highest weight last year. I should feel victorious, and I do, but I also feel sad and overwhelmed by my puppy issues.

The trainer episode about did me in. I had Greg pick up Kip Christmas eve (they made us wait till 9 p.m.); what I saw made me want to cry. My dog has lost an incredible amount of weight for such a short time, was fearful and snappy. Here his pictured at left, drinking half this bucket of water Christmas eve; his sister is at right; they used to be the same width before the training. A healthy weight.

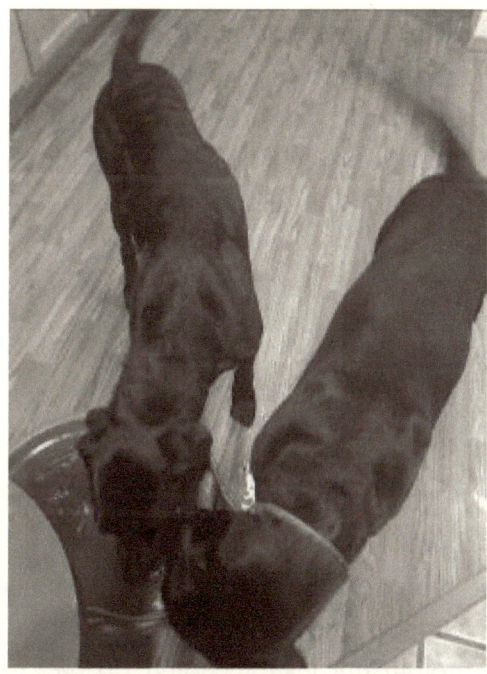

It took everything I had to send him back for the last few days of training after keeping him 2.5 days. He has come back more aggressive and no longer as cuddly. He hasn't slept in my arms yet, which he did before (every night) for the last 13 months. He snapped my leg three times when a dog charged him at the vet's (no puncture wound), and he got in a fight with Miza and bit his sister, both of which he has never done before. So much for the dang training. He also, in trying to run away from the trainer (both times I "visited" he succeeded), learned to jump fences, so now I have that additional worry.

So year ahead? Missions? Goals?

Clearly, I'm afraid to walk him, but I must.

The trainer says he must learn to bond with Greg, but Greg is not one who seems to want to bond with him. I am at a loss.

In any case, I don't want to leave you hanging while I'm hanging in confusion-upset land, when I should be happy and proud of all I've accomplished, so I'll give this diary one more week, so it's an actual year from my start date of January 7, 2015.

In the meantime, the good news is that I've learned I can control my weight and my eating without writing everything down every day; I've learned what works for me and what doesn't, and as you can see, I haven't been writing down my weight or exercise for the last 11 days (too traumatized worrying about and missing Kip), yet I've managed to lose over 3 pounds. So that's good.

January 1 – January 4

Weight: 155.6
Exercise: Averaged 7,300 steps

Hope

Saw "my" psychiatrist today, the one who put me on Zoloft about 6 weeks ago, for my anxiety. (By the way, I never went to a psychiatrist for pills; I don't really know what happened. First minute, I was taking my family to "family counseling" because it was available through my insurance and I'd met my deductibles; next thing I know, I'm being prescribed SSRIs by her partner, a psychiatrist. Weird. Hate to think a "health care" place would be dastardly, but I wonder if it was so the clinic could make more money?)

Because I've plummeted into a major depression since I started the pills, along with lack of energy, stomach issues, battling weight gain (therefore having to drop my food intake even more), he instantly saw I had a problem and took me off the medication. Thank God. I'm not saying it won't help some people, but it clearly put me into a spin into despair. It didn't help that the increase in the prescription coincided with my dog going to the trainer's, which made me more anxious and depressed than ever. Now he's switching me to Buspar, focusing on the anxiety only.

"Before I came here to see you," I said, "I didn't have depression. Yes, I worry too much, and I have anxiety issues, all increased when I quit smoking and milk chocolate, which were my personal self-medications, and both of which I will never go back to again. But now I'm depressed, really depressed."

"You're definitely having a bad reaction to the medication. We're taking you off it now."

You think?

I'm hesitant to try another drug, but I'll give old Buspar a month's try, maybe starting tomorrow. It would be nice not to be hyper-worrying (anxious) so much. I didn't realize how much cigarettes were a "therapy" of sorts for me. They are also murderous little cancer sticks, so I never want to go back there.

Yesterday, everything felt hopeless. I felt hopeless, mainly because of Kip and his issues, and that it seemed I could never walk my dogs freely in the woods again…which means my health and sanity will suffer, as that is the best part of my day. The only time my head is cleared of all garbage and worries (except now I have to worry about Kip pulling a move against a dog charging toward him).

Today seems better. Greg is building a smaller, taller fenced area, which is not easy in the frozen land, that Kip can't jump (since he learned to jump fences trying to escape the trainer). That will relieve a lot of my anxiety right there. And sneaking away for a walk, far from people or trails, this morning, where I know no other people go (only moose), was awesome. And getting off the dang drug that is making me tumble into darkness is good too.

Yesterday was bleak. Today I have hope. And I can write again.

January 5, Tuesday

Weight: 155.3
Ate: 2 Amy's meals, ½ cup peanuts, smoothie, dark-chocolate covered walnuts and raisins
Exercise: Dog walk: 10,437 steps

TOPS First Weigh-in of the Year

I'm a KOPS now. I can gain 3 pounds or lose 7 and still stay in KOPS status. (I wish I could worry about losing 7! Ha!). I "made" KOPS at 154; today I'm 155.3, yet still I dare to wear jeans (because they look good and are a size 6; can you believe it? Of course, they are the D2G jeans with the stretchy waist, but I'll take it.) So I throw them on and a shirt, and suddenly I've gained 2.5 pounds. Should still be good for the TOPS weigh-in.

January 6, Wednesday

Weight: 154.2
Ate: 2 Amy's burritos, vegan burger with fries and veggies, ½ cup peanuts
Exercise: Dog walk: 11,169 steps

Feeling Better

Without the Zoloft, having been switched to Buspar (for anxiety), plus of course with Kip home from the trainer, the depression has lifted. I feel hopeful again. I had tumbled me into bleakness, but I've crawled out, and made my step goal the last 3 days and walked the dogs again. So if you end up being medicated by a psychiatrist, like I was the last 6 weeks, and the medication doesn't feel right, know yourself, take a stand. Fortunately, by the one-month check in with him a few days ago, he was immediately able to see that the medication was wrong for me (even though I sensed it early on). I'm not saying Zoloft won't help some people, but it sure made me feel worse. I'm back!

January 7, Thursday

Weight: 154
Exercise: 12,481 steps
Inches: Chest: 40.5 Waist: 34.75 Hips: 39.9
Body Fat %: 27.11 BMI: 26-3/7

Statistics for the Year

In one year, I have lost 56 pounds (and don't forget...quit smoking!). I lost 39 inches in the following areas measured in the past year:

- Chest: 9.5
- Waist: 10.5
- Hips: 10.2
- Wrist (left): 0.75
- Forearm (left): 1.05
- Thigh (left): 4.25
- Upper Arm (right): 2.75

My lean body weight has reduced from 149.75 to 112.25; my body fat weight has gone from 60.25 to 41.75; my body fat % has decreased from 28.69 to 27.11. My BMI was at a morbidly obese 36 on January 7 a year ago and is slightly above normal at 26-3/7 today (a loss of 4 more pounds, which I have no doubt I will achieve this year, will bring me into normal BMI!). This all without any major "dieting" or starvation, or any excess exercise...mostly just a 45-minute dog walk a day and some additional housecleaning and walking to aim for 10,000 steps most days the past few months. I dropped from XXL stretch pants to size 6 jeans with some stretch to them, size 8 and 10 with no stretch. I went from 2X shirts (tight) to size medium (fit fine). Wow! Proud of me!

Most of all, I did it without going too "hangry" (hungry and angry). The smoothies seemed to fill me up. I didn't use diet pills, and the only supplements I ended up using, after trying various ones, were a vitamin B12 every other day (since I'm vegan).

I am stronger, fitter, and look better than I have in years. I achieved KOPS status at TOPS. I'm good. Sigh.

One Year

So I made it a year, but I feel that I've made a lifelong commitment to better health and change, so the milestone is rather meaningless. I know I will continue to eat simply, small meals, vegan. I know I will continue to take walks in the woods, and maybe, when it's too icy, on a treadmill or around the house. I will continue to be a nonsmoker.

Now that I've reached my weight loss goal, are my "goals" over? Well, not really. I love the feeling of being "done," but I expect to continue to work on strengthening my muscles, conquering my anxiety, and training my fearful dog. So, life is filled with challenges and adventures ahead. Mostly, I want to learn to be at peace more, and happier more, so with this in mind, I have started listening to a meditation app and researching ways to bring peace and happiness into my life more often.

What I Did Right and Wrong This *Year*

What I have done right is:

- I lost weight, inches, BMI. I reached my goal. It wasn't my initial goal (4 pounds over it), but I'm okay with that. My body stopped when it needed to. Perhaps I'll lose a few more pounds this year, and step into the 140s, but I'll just keep doing what I'm doing. No worries.
- I quit smoking May 14. I slowly gave up most unhealthy foods and drinks, including cutting back to one Diet Coke a

week and almost no sugar.

- I still allow myself a taste of chocolate nearly every day. I don't feel deprived.
- I made a commitment to helping animals by going vegan, and this is a lifetime change. I feel great about this. It also made losing weight so much easier.
- I journaled almost daily. When I stopped journaling daily, the last few weeks (both overwhelmed with fears about my puppy at what I considered unkind training and on prescribed medication that made me feel much worse), I still stayed with my diet and continued to lose or maintain my weight.
- I learned to use and love my Fitbit. I aimed for 10,000 steps a day and achieved that most days since I got the Fitbit last fall.
- As a vegetarian who hated vegetables, I learned to incorporate them into my daily diet, especially through my smoothies, soups, and Amy's Kitchen frozen meals.
- I modeled for my son that a commitment to health and wellness can work. A year ago I smoked and was morbidly obese. Today I am fit and healthy *and* a nonsmoker.

What I have done wrong is:

- I made mistakes, I'm sure, but I'm happy with my progress. I feel good, and I forgive any errors I've made. Overall, I stuck with the diet, I learned to eat less (especially less fattening foods and more fruits and vegetables) and exercise a little bit more (especially after getting a Fitbit and striving for 10,000 steps a day). I haven't learned to love or even go to the gym yet, and I'd like to do that, but perhaps that is just not and never will be me. And I'm okay with that. If I'm happiest on the trails with my dog, who is to criticize? It seems that the most critical person of me is me. I'll let it go. If it happens, it happens, and if it doesn't, *que sera sera*. Life does go on, thankfully, and I'll be grateful for every day I have left. Especially now that I'm in size 6 (stretch) and size 8 (no stretch) jeans!

FINAL THOUGHTS

Thank you for sharing my weight-loss journey with me. I wish you the best on your own journey.

For me, the new year came and passed, and I was, like a year ago on January 1, without resolutions. But somehow, a week after the new year arrived, an idea came to me. Just like a year ago I decided to lose weight (and how that journey became so much more as I learned to live a healthy lifestyle!), this year I find myself committing to improving my mental (anxiety) and spiritual self.

Just like with my weight loss and quitting smoking, I will begin by watching relevant documentaries, immersing myself in books and articles, downloading apps, talking with others, and most importantly, exploring my own transformation through a personal journal. I stopped taking the Buspar, by the way, which suddenly started giving me "brain zaps" (sort of like an electric shock to the brain), and decided to work to solve my anxiety issues just as I have my weight and smoking issues, using the same techniques of self-education and personal study of what works best for me.

It is exciting to have found a new goal in bettering myself. I am excited for *you*, too! Losing weight was not always easy, not always fun, but overall it was well worth it. I learned to care about my own body and my health in a way I have never done before in my 55 years. It helped me to know you, my readers, were out there, rooting for me, hoping for the best. I may not know you personally (like you now know me), but I feel like we have been through so much together. This has been a year of victories and joy, as well as of loss (dear Chewie), anxiety, and fear (especially regarding my poor scared pup, Kip). The yin and the yang, perhaps.

And such is life.

It goes on. And because of my weight loss journey, I feel like mine might go on a little longer, a lot stronger, and certainly happier. Best of luck to you, and thank you for being such an integral part of my journey!

EPILOGUE

What My Dogs Have Taught Me about Weight Loss

I struggled with weight, up and down, repeatedly. But one day I decided to put away the diet books and stop watching weight-loss videos and instead pay attention to what my dogs were teaching me. This is what I learned.

One large meal a day is enough, and it's best to spread it out into two small meals. That way you're not too hungry.

Snacks and treats are fine, but you must work for them. But that's okay, because work is fun!

You can keep things simple. You don't have to eat a wide variety of foods all the time. Find what food choices work for you, keep you healthy, and stick with them.

Exercise is *always* fun, especially when you're with a friend.

You don't need a gym membership to lose weight. We will never turn down a stroll in the woods, a run through a field, or even just exploring the yard.

Rides in cars are interesting, but it's always better to walk if you can.

As we age, we need less food.

Some of us have different metabolisms than others. We can't all eat the same amount or the same types of foods and expect to weigh the same. So adjust the food for your body's needs.

There are certain foods you should just never eat if you don't want to be fat or unhealthy. Once you accept that is the rule, things are easier.

Every day, no matter how you feel or how much pain you are in, you will feel better if you take a walk. Even a short walk is better than none.

When you're young, it's fun to run, but it turns out walking is just fine. It turns out you can lose a lot of weight by just walking a little bit every day.

Some of us can't walk as fast or as far as others. But we still enjoy a walk.

It's okay to rest during walks if you need it.

Obesity can shorten our lives. Like people, obesity in pets can cause diabetes, joint disease, heart disease, liver disease, skin disease, respiratory disease, heat stroke, and even cancer.

We might act like we want treats all the time, but we don't need them to be happy.

We take great joy in walks, but we also love relaxation time, massages, and sleep, and we don't feel guilty when it's time to stop exercising or if we want to take a day off.

Drink lots of water. Always have some available – in the car, on your hikes, in the house – wherever you are. Water keeps us alive. Water helps us not be too hungry.

Finally, we come in all shapes, sizes, and types. Take joy in your body, your loved ones, your life, just as you are. The least of our worries is how we look to others. There is so much more to life. The simple, smallest things are what matter, not whether you're a collie or a bulldog, a St. Bernard or a beagle, or a mutt.

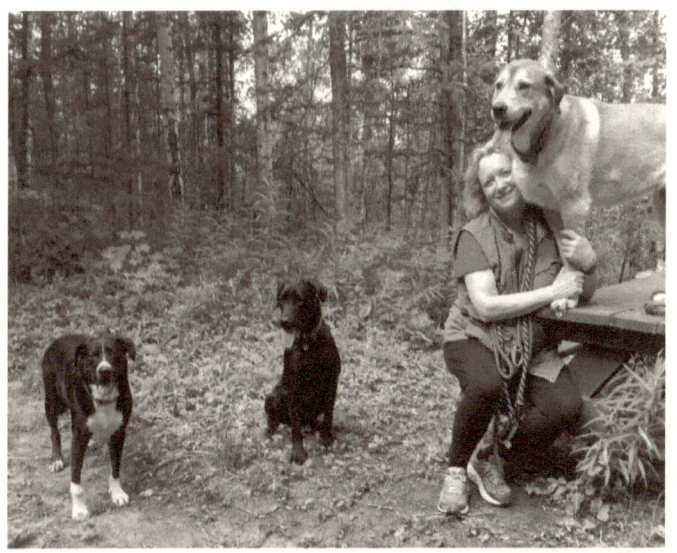

WORKS CITED

Arbour, Nicole. "Dear Fat People." *YouTube.com*. September 3, 2015. Website accessed September 14, 2015: https://www.youtube.com/watch?v=CXFgNhyP4-A

Arcade Fire. "My Body Is a Cage." *Neon Bible* (album). Merge Records: 2007.

Chutkan, Robynne. "What Your Stool Is Telling You." DoctorOz.com. September 14, 2011. Website accessed September 24, 2015: http://www.doctoroz.com/article/what-your-stool-telling-you?page=2

"Dr. Oz's 5-Day Summer Cleanse." Dr. Oz Show. July 13, 2015. Web site accessed July 14, 2015: http://www.doctoroz.com/article/dr-ozs-5-day-summer-cleanse

"Easy Summer Cleanse." The Dr. Oz Show. July 13, 2015. Web site accessed July 14, 2015: http://www.doctoroz.com/episode/easy-summer-cleanse

Edwards, Ros (director). *Autopsy: The Last Hours of: Elvis Presley*. (*Autopsy: The Last Hours:* Season 3, Episode 1). December 2, 2014.

Fat, Sick & Nearly Dead. A Joe Gross Film. Director: Joe Gross. April 1, 2011.

Fat, Sick & Nearly Dead 2. A Joe Gross Film. Director: Kurt Engfehr. September 18, 2014.

HealthyWage Blog. "Where Do I Start? Advice from HealthyWage Participants: Volume 2." Healthywage.com. Website accessed August 25, 2015: https://healthywage.wordpress.com/2013/04/05/where-do-i-start-advice-from-healthywage-participants-volume-2/

HBO Films. *The Weight of the Nation: The Quest to Understand the Biology of Weight Loss*. Executive Producers Sheila Nevins, John Hoffman. 2012. Web site accessed July 13, 2015: http://theweightofthenation.hbo.com/films/bonus-shorts/the-quest-to-understand-the-biology-of-weight-loss

Helwick, Caroline. "Vast Majority of Hoarders Overweight or Obese." *Medscape*. March 28, 2011. Web site accessed July 27, 2015: http://www.medscape.com/viewarticle/739795

"New research shows link between obesity and hoarding." *HubPages*. May 4, 2014. Web site accessed July 27, 2015: http://bje117.hubpages.com/hub/Your-body-is-a-temple-not-a-store-house-ten-tips-to-lose-the-weight-and-the-clutter-in-your-life

"Guided Reboot." *Reboot with Joe*. Web site accessed August 1, 2015: http://www.rebootwithjoe.com/rebooting/guided-reboot/

Medical Bag. "Elvis Presley." *Features: What Killed 'Em*. August 13, 2012. Website accessed September 24, 2015: https://www.themedicalbag.com/story/elvis-presley

Mitchell, Andie. *Weight-Loss Win*. Website accessed November 14, 2015: https://www.yahoo.com/health/tagged/weight-loss-win

Newley, Anthony, and Leslie Bricusse. "Feeling Good." Song from the musical *The Roar of the Greasepaint – The Smell of the Crowd*. 1964. Recorded by Nina Simone. YouTube channel accessed August 23, 2015: https://www.youtube.com/watch?v=w8_5MLtlBEE&list=PLYFeVqKDpxwrgOYtLn5fLWzsreS-9WVDs&index=3

"Scientists Find Link Between Dopamine and Obesity." Brookhaven National Laboratory. February 1, 2001. Web site accessed July 27, 2015: https://www.bnl.gov/bnlweb/pubaf/pr/2001/bnlpr020101.htm

Simon, Carly. "Attitude Dancing." *Playing Possum*. Album. 1975.

"Symptoms of Hyperparathyroidism." *Parathyroid.com*. Web site accessed July 29, 2015: http://www.parathyroid.com/parathyroid-symptoms.htm

"Symptoms of Hypoparathyroidism." *Hypoparathyroidism.com*. Web site accessed July 29, 2015: http://hypoparathyroidism.com/symptoms-of-hypoparathyroidism/

Watson, Erica. "It Ain't Over Until the Black Fat Lady Sings: Dear Nicole Arbour, Fat Shaming IS a Thing." *The Blog*. Ebony.com. September 11, 2015. Website accessed September

14, 2015: http://www.huffingtonpost.com/ebonycom/it-aint-over-until-the-bl_b_8122848.html

White Ink, online reviewer. IMDB.com. *The Weight of the Nation: The Quest to Understand the Biology of Weight Loss.* Web site accessed July 13, 2015: http://www.imdb.com/title/tt2689766/

Wurtman, Judith J. "Serotonin: What It is and Why It's Important for Weight Loss." *Psychology Today.com.* Web site accessed July 27, 2015: https://www.psychologytoday.com/blog/the-antidepressant-diet/201008/serotonin-what-it-is-and-why-its-important-weight-loss

Wylde, Bryce. "The Dopamine Diet." *The Dr. Oz Show.* May 10, 2013. Web site accessed July 27, 2015: http://www.doctoroz.com/article/dopamine-diet?page=1

ABOUT THE AUTHOR

Jory Ames writes and lives in Alaska. She has lived throughout the Northwest and taught English for 18 years. She enjoys her family, writing, reading, music, nature hikes, mountains, dogs, and cats but is not so much a fan of cold Alaskan winters. Jory has been volunteering for humane societies since 1977, particularly focusing on ending pet overpopulation and the killing of healthy, adoptable dogs and cats at animal control shelters. She has published hundreds of poems, short stories, articles, and essays in newspapers, literary journals, and magazines. She is especially grateful to her readers.

WORKS BY JORY AMES

NONFICTION
Birth 101: Reflections of a Reluctant Mother
For the Love of Dogs: My Life in Dog Years
Poor Little Allison: The Struggle to Survive a Loved One's Murder
Weight Loss Diary with Food & Exercise Journal: 16 Weeks to a Better Body
Weight Loss Journey: Changing My Life, One Pound and Story at a Time
Weight Loss Journey: Part Two: Reaching Goal, One Pound and Story at a Time

POETRY
Lucifer and Other Love Poems
Poems of Love, Loss, and Regret

CONTACT THE AUTHOR:

I appreciate your reading my book. Here is how you can contact me:

E-mail: joryames@gmail.com